Occlusion and Restorative Dentistry for the General Practitioner

Occlusion and Restorative Dentistry for the General Practitioner

Michael D. Wise
MScD, BDS, FDS

1986

BDJ

Published by the British Dental Association
64 Wimpole Street, London W1M 8AL

British Library Cataloguing in Publication Data

Wise, Michael D.
Occlusion and restorative dentistry for
general practitioner.—2nd ed.
1. Occlusion (Dentistry)
I. Title
617.6′43   RK523
ISBN 0–904588–12–2

Typeset, printed and bound in Great Britain by
Latimer Trend and Company Ltd, Plymouth

Foreword

This book contains the ten articles that were published as a series in the *British Dental Journal* from February 16 to July 6, 1982. My aim was to present a practical approach to occlusion in restorative dentistry. It was inevitable that there was a limit on space so the anatomical and physiological details have been omitted.

It is my firm conviction that if a restorative dental practice is to be run in a controlled and predictable manner, the dentist must have a sound background in periodontics, operative dentistry, endodontics, occlusion and laboratory techniques. However, we all know that it is one thing to read articles and attend lectures, but quite another to apply the knowledge. I hope that the concepts contained in this book will stimulate you to form study clubs so that together you can explore occlusion and laboratory techniques further, and then apply them to your practice.

Acknowledgements

I would like to express my sincere thanks to Mr W. M. Tay, who has given invaluable assistance in editing the manuscripts, also to Mr W. J. Morgan and his photographic department at the Institute of Dental Surgery, Eastman Dental Hospital, and in particular to Mr A. P. Johnson. I am grateful for the help of Mr B. J. Parkins and Mr D. J. Setchell, with whom I teach the occlusion course at the Institute of Dental Surgery. I also thank Professor G. A. Morrant, who has encouraged the teaching of occlusion in his department, Mrs S. R. Morgan for typing the manuscript, Mr A. Laurie, whose technical work is shown in the majority of the clinical photographs, and the Cordent Dental Trust which has given financial assistance with the colour reproductions.

I would also like to take this opportunity to express my gratitude to Miss M. A. Clennett for assistance with the references, Professor A. G. Alexander for his support, my patients who have allowed me to take photographs, and my wife, Priscilla, who has encouraged many long hours of writing.

Contents

1 Preliminary Considerations and Examination Procedures

Preliminary considerations

The current usage of the term 'occlusion' embraces three major areas of dentistry namely: the basic science, that is, the anatomy and physiology of the masticatory system; clinical and animal research (associated principally with periodontitis and tooth mobility, temporomandibular joint dysfunction and the investigation of clinical techniques); and its clinical application, which is the management of the occlusion in daily practice, and is as important in a simple occlusal amalgam as in full mouth rehabilitation.

Many of the theories and philosophies of occlusion have been developed from experience by conscientious practitioners, and some of these concepts are now being investigated scientifically, although owing to difficulties in clinical research, there is still a lack of knowledge and good publications. Furthermore, it is not always possible to relate the findings of the experimental studies directly to clinical practice. At the time of writing, most of the clinical philosophies remain untested and can be challenged readily for their empirical nature.

The conscientious practitioner, therefore, is in a dilemma. He needs guidelines to assist him with the multitude of occlusal problems with which he is faced daily. He cannot wait for the researchers to produce the data before he restores the ravages of dental disease. This series of articles is designed to fill this need.

The dentist should realise that most of the responses to occlusal disharmonies are adaptive in nature, that is changes may occur in the masticatory apparatus in an effort to relieve the disharmony. For example, teeth may wear, become mobile or drift; jaw muscles may alter the paths of

1

mandibular movement, and the mandibular condyle may, as a result of altered muscle activity, adopt a new relationship to the disc and fossa.

The following should be considered whenever the occlusal surface is to be involved in a restoration:

The 'high' restoration

The possibility of converting a patient with a symptom-free adapting occlusion to one who is uncomfortable because of high fillings increases with the number and complexity of the restorations. Furthermore, the response varies between individuals and within the same individual, owing to central mechanisms which affect tolerance. The dentist should be aware of the diagnostic criteria and clinical techniques which allow him to plan a sequence of treatment predictably, thereby obviating the need for prolonged sessions of grinding-in restorations and/or unnecessary conflict with the dental technician.

Mechanical failure of restorations

Restorations can fail mechanically through:

Fracture of restorative material (such as amalgam or porcelain); of a remaining tooth; or of joints in fixed bridge work.

Cementation failure owing to stress concentration in the cement or owing to flexion or wear of restoration margins resulting in exposure and rapid dissolution of the cement.

Wear When a patient presents with mechanical failure of restorations the dentist must find out its cause, whether or not it be inadequate tooth preparation, unsatisfactory manipulation of the restorative materials and/ or the result of occlusal disharmonies.

When he plans a restoration he must know how to direct occlusal stresses favourably through the tooth and restorative material. (See Chapter 6.)

Attrition

Occlusal wear is compensated for by adaptive mechanisms.[1] However, compensation may not be complete, so that with severe attrition there may be loss of occlusal vertical dimension[2] and with minimal attrition there may be an increase in vertical face height.[3] If restorations are required, the complication of differential wear is introduced.

Differential wear

Dental materials wear at different rates, and none of the currently available materials simulates the wear of enamel or dentine. Therefore unequal wear can take place where restorations oppose intact tooth surfaces or restorations of dissimilar material (fig. 1.1).

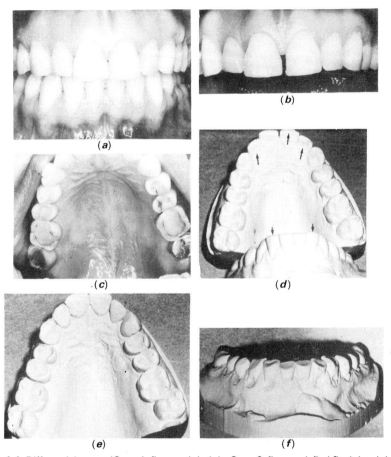

Fig 1.1 Differential wear (Case 1 figures (*a*)–(*c*). Case 2 figures (*d*)–(*f*): (*a*) original alignment of 321|123; (*b*) two years later; (*c*) worn occlusal composite restorations. The composites were placed by the patient's dentist after fig 1.1 (*a*). Excessive posterior wear has resulted in heavy contact between 321|123 and 321|123 and subsequent movement of 21|12 to relieve the load, that is, and adaptation. (*d*) The patient complained of wear 321|123 and drifting of 1|1 No wear on 321|123. The dentist provided PJCs for 321|123; (*e*) Upper cast 6 years later. (*f*) Lower cast 6 years later. Note the wear, which is aesthetically unacceptable to the patient.

Bruxism

The spontaneous or subconscious gnashing or grinding of teeth can, according to some authors be precipitated by occlusal disharmonies and as such can be eliminated by occlusal adjustment.[4] The evidence for this is sparse. In bruxism, the problems associated with high restorations, mechanical failure and differential wear become heightened. The dentist should design the occlusal surfaces of restorations so as to reduce these problems. In figure 1.2(*a*) the restoration on 3| was satisfactory for 10 years but became uncemented shortly after placement of a large bonded porcelain crown |6 (fig. 1.2(*b*)). Owing to this crown being high, the patient found her grinding habit becoming worse. Her grinding on |6 and |6 also resulted in contact between 3| and 3| (fig. 1.2(*c*)). Replacement temporary crowns for 3| were unsuccessful, and the problem was only cured by occlusal adjustment of |6. Although this did not stop her bruxing completely, the interference removed from the |6 altered the pattern so as to obviate the adverse mechanical effects on the 3|. Subsequently a new crown was provided for |6.

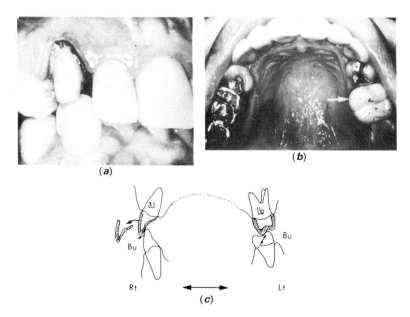

(*a*) (*b*) (*c*)

Fig. 1.2(*a*) 3| uncemented after 10 years. (*b*) Large bonded crown on |6. This was high particularly in lateral excursion (3| temporarily recemented). (*c*) Frontal view (Bu=buccal, Lt=patient's left, Rt=patient's right) showing right lateral excursion. Bruxism on |6 and |6 resulted in contact of 3| and 3| and cementation failure of 3|. Arrows indicate the direction of mandibular movement during bruxism (see text).

Drifting of anterior teeth

A forward positioning of the mandible in an attempt to avoid posterior occlusal disharmonies may result in labial movement of the upper incisors through the force applied by the lower incisors (figs 1.3(*a*) and (*b*)). This movement is particularly liable to occur with teeth affected by periodontitis.

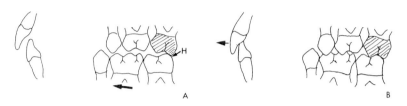

Fig. 1.3 Sagittal view. (*a*) Crown on |7 is high. One adaptive possibility is for the path of closure to alter so as to avoid the high spot H (fig. 3(*b*)). This may result in 21|12 and 21|12 contacting, with subsequent labial movement of 21|12.

Mobility

There are three situations in which occlusal loads can increase tooth mobility.

(1) 'Normal' periodontium and increased loads, for example in bruxism (fig. 1.4(*a*)).
(2) Periodontitis and 'normal' or increased load (fig. 4(*b*)).
(3) Reduced but healthy periodontium (that is following correction of periodontitis or shortening of a root, for example apicectomy) and 'normal' load (fig. 1.4(*c*)).

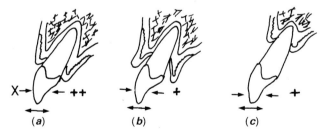

Fig. 1.4(*a*) 'Normal' but widened periodontium with increased load + + = increased mobility but no loss of attachment X = effect of circumoral musculature. (*b*) Periodontitis: increased mobility may be due to inflammation and/or loss of support and/or increased occlusal load. (*c*) Reduced periodontium: a tooth with a reduced but healthy periodontium may have increased mobility.

The practitioner must recognise these conditions and know when therapy is required. It is important to note that mobility is a sign not a disease.

Periodontitis

The periodontium is the foundation of restorative dentistry. The effect of excessive occlusal forces on the progression of periodontitis is still unresolved. Some authors believe that these factors can accelerate the rate of breakdown in the presence of plaque and established periodontitis. However, others consider these occlusal factors to be insignificant (see bibliography).

Stability

Assuming that occlusal factors are important, the dentist must decide whether he is able to achieve occlusal stability in an adjusted or restored dentition. If stability is not possible, is the practitioner able to control subsequent occlusal changes so as to prevent the detrimental effects of developing disharmonies?

Temporomandibular joints and muscles

The influence of occlusion on these structures is twofold:
(1) Whether or not discrepancies in the occlusion resulting from restorative dentistry can precipitate temporomandibular joint (TMJ) dysfunction.
(2) Whether or not the patient with established TMJ dysfunction requires special precautions in restorative dentistry.

Some authors report that occlusal factors can precipitate TMJ pain and dysfunction in the susceptible patient[5] and that patients with established pain require careful handling of their occlusion when restorations are required so as not to exacerbate their symptoms.

Having considered briefly the major areas of concern regarding the occlusion it is prudent to consider:

The occlusal examination for patients requiring restorative therapy

The equipment needed is:

Chart

A charting system must incorporate the following: history, periodontal chart, mobility chart, extra-oral examination, intra-oral examination, and radiographic report.

Some practitioners may prefer to see sections arranged as check-off lists. However, the author prefers to leave spaces under major headings, to give flexibility of charting.

Tray set-up for occlusal examination

A basic set-up (fig. 1.5) consists of: mouth mirror; face mirror for patient; periodontal probe (Marquis with 3 mm colour coding*); occlusal articulating paper—blue; occlusal tape—black, red and green held in Millers forceps; shimstock 12µm plastic foil (a convenient substitute can be made easily by feeding a proprietory 'space blanket' (Thermos) obtained from the chemist, into an office paper shredder. Prior to placement in the shredder, the backing is removed from the silver foil and the foil placed between sheets of A4 paper. The resulting strips may be cut into 5 mm lengths and used as shims[6]); Mosquito forceps for holding shimstock; 2 × 2 inch gauze or medical wipes (Kleenex).

History-taking and examination

There are four essentials: history-taking, extra-oral examination, intra-oral

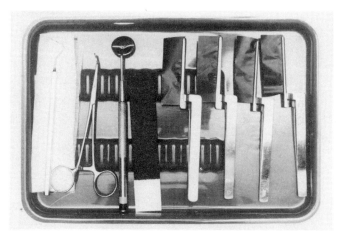

Fig 1.5 Tray set up for an occlusal examination. (*Left to right*) Gauze with Marquis probe, shimstock in mosquito forceps, mouth mirror, thick articulating paper, occlusal tape in forceps×4 (one black, two red, one green).

---

*Details will be found at the end of each chapter.

examination, special investigation, such as study casts, diagnostic wax-ups, and pantographic surveys.

All new and recall patients should have their occlusions examined. Dentists should develop a 'graded examination procedure' the extent of examination being determined by the patient's restorative requirements. For example, the 22-year-old (on routine recall) with a past history of minimal caries requires a less thorough examination than the patient presenting with advanced periodontitis, missing teeth and large restorations, and who is obviously destined for extensive therapy if the dentition is to be salvaged.

The relative sparsity of clinical studies accounts for present occlusal diagnostic criteria being somewhat subjective. It is a combination of various signs and symptoms which gives the indication of occlusal problems, more than the presence of a single factor. It must be remembered that many dentitions which have malaligned or missing teeth are functionally acceptable (fig. 1.6).

The following examination procedure is that used by the author for a patient requiring restorative care, rather than one with TMJ pain-dysfunction syndrome. The reader is advised to refer to Zarb and Carlsson, *TMJ Function and Dysfunction* for an account of the latter.

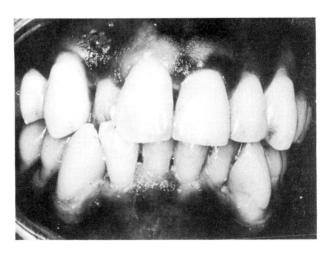

Fig. 1.6 Dentition of 60-year-old. Although 2| and 2̄| are in 'crossbite' there is no mobility, no drifting, no pocketing, no TMJ disturbance or problems with mastication. The malocclusion is functionally acceptable.

History

Record the main complaint, that is, the reason for the patient's attendance. Is the patient aware of:

- Pain in the joints or associated muscle areas?
- Clicking or locking of the joints?
- Rubbing or grinding of the teeth (frequent complaints by patient's spouse or room-mate)?
- Oral habits such as pencil or lip sucking?
- Looseness of teeth?
- Movement of teeth, particularly the upper anterior segments?
- Pain in the teeth?
- Repeated fractures of restorations or teeth, cementation failures of bridge work?

Extra-oral examination

The areas to be examined are the temporomandibular joints and the muscles of mastication.

The patient should be placed in a semi-reclining position in the dental chair with his head properly supported.

Temporomandibular joints　The joints are palpated anterior to the external auditory meati, and the patient is asked to open and close the jaws. Note any crepitus, limitation of movement, pain on movement, or lateral deviation.

Muscles of mastication: palpation　Temporalis and masseter muscles

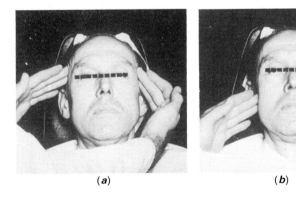

(a)　　　　　　　　　　(b)

Fig. 1.7 Palpation of (*a*) temporalis and (*b*) masseter muscles (note the larger left masseter).

should be palpated as in figure 1.7 in the resting and clenched state. Pain may be elicited from these muscles which may be symptomless otherwise.

Spontaneous contraction   While the patient is sitting in the chair observe carefully any contraction of the masseter muscles. This is probably brought on by the stress of the dental visit and is an indication of an insidious bruxing habit.[7]

Intra-oral examination
This includes: muscles, teeth, periodontium, radiographs and occlusal relationships.

Muscles   Three muscles are examined on each side: lateral pterygoid, medial pterygoid and temporalis.

Lateral pterygoid   The patient is asked to open slightly and move the jaw towards the side to be palpated, that is right lateral pterygoid move to the right. The finger of the operator is then slid along the anterior ramus of the mandible and up behind the tuberosity (figs 1.8(*a*) and (*b*)). Lateral pterygoid tenderness is usually demonstrated by the patient screwing up the eyes with discomfort or moving the head away from the examining finger.

(One publication suggests that the above procedure stimulates a trigger area associated with the insertion of the temporalis muscle and not the lateral pterygoid muscle.[8])

Medial pterygoid   The patient should open as wide as possible and the index finger should be slid along the anterior border of the ascending ramus

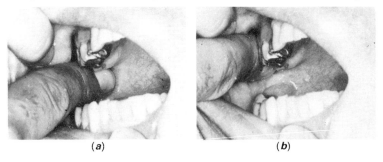

(*a*)   (*b*)

Fig. 1.8 Palpation of trigger point in the region of the lateral pterygoid muscle. (*a*) Positioning finger. (*b*) Palpation behind the tuberosity.

to the level of the hamular notch, and then the tip of the finger moved approximately 1 cm medially towards the uvula. Pressure is then applied laterally, and if tender a similar response to lateral pterygoid tenderness is elicited.

Insertion of temporalis is palpated on the anterior border of the ascending ramus and may elicit tenderness.

Teeth and periodontium   Patients exhibiting symptoms and signs of occlusal disturbances in the teeth and periodontium, can be broadly divided into two groups: Group A are resistant to periodontitis and generally have pale pink, thick gingivae and shallow crevices. These are so-called wear patients (fig. 1.9); Group B are susceptible to periodontitis (fig. 1.10).

It is essential to bear these groups in mind during the examination and be aware that there are patients who may show intermediate features of these extremes.

The following should be recorded: teeth present, pocket depths and bleeding, mobility, tooth positions and tooth crowns.

The teeth present should be charted at both initial and subsequent recall examinations. Crevice depth measurements at the mesial, middle and distal thirds of the buccal and lingual aspects of each tooth should be made and recorded when over 3 mm deep. A record should be made of bleeding points and used as an index of inflammation.

Each tooth should be tested for mobility (fig. 1.11). Apply the handle of a

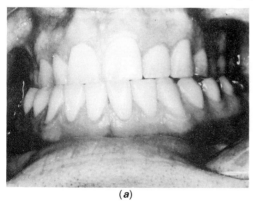

(a)

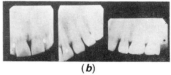

(b)

Fig. 1.9(a) 35-year-old patient exhibiting wear. Note thick firm pink gingivae and worn incisal edges. (b) Note dense high interdental bone and worn crowns

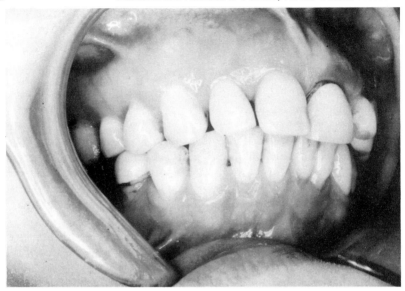

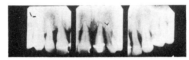

Fig. 1.10 (*Top*) 35-year-old patient who is susceptible to periodontitis; (*bottom*) note bone loss.

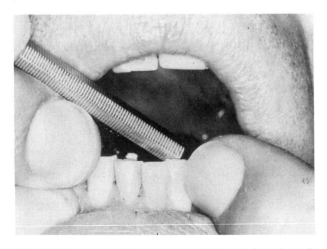

Fig. 1.11 Testing mobility: mirror handle lingual, finger buccal.

dental mirror to one aspect of the tooth crown and with the examining finger of the other hand placed on the other aspect, a subjective assessment of the degree of mobility is made. It is important that mobility be recorded on a charting system for subsequent review, for unless the dentist has previous records, he would not know whether mobility is increasing or decreasing. None of the current indices makes this assessment entirely reliable; however, a useful recording system is that described by Schluger et al.[9] as follows. Movement is estimated and scored from 1 to 3 with half increments marked as (+). Interpretation of the values is:

0—normal mobility less than 1 mm
1—mobility approximately 1 mm buccolingually
2—mobility 2 mm buccolingually but nil in an apical direction
3—mobility greater than 2 mm buccolingually and apical movement.

However, a mobile tooth may move out of the way when the patient closes, and it is valuable to know if this is occurring. This is tested as in figures 1.12(a) and (b) (fremitus).

Diastemata, particularly of anterior teeth, migration of teeth, over-erupted and tilted teeth should be noted. These are best observed on study casts (fig. 1.13).

The following features of the tooth crowns should be noted: wear (distribution and degree of faceting), chipped and fractured cusps, fractured restorations, uncemented bridges and micro-cracks in enamel (fig. 1.14).

Facets should be matched on opposing teeth, and the patient may be asked to move the jaw into such a position. Some patients may express incredulity at the eccentric locations of the facets and may initially experience difficulty in positioning the jaws. However, this is easily

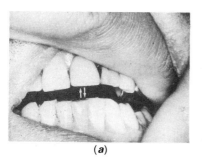
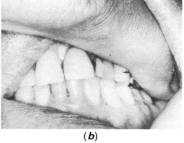

(a)   (b)

Fig. 1.12 Testing for fremitus. (a) The forefinger is placed on the labial surfaces of the upper teeth and the patient guided to tap his teeth together. (b) Movement of upper teeth can be detected by the palpating finger.

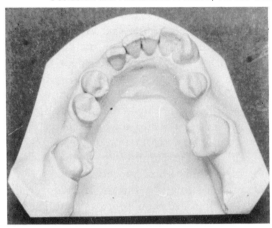

Fig. 1.13 Study casts showing migration, tilting, spaces and crowding.

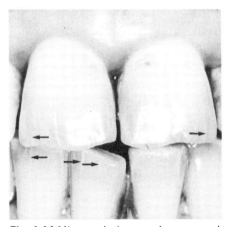

Fig. 1.14 Microcracks in enamel are arrowed.

overcome by using a face mirror and appropriate guidance from the operator. When a scooped-out facet is present on a restoration the relationship of the opposing cusp should also be noted, that is whether or not it has overerupted into the facet. This is especially important if the restoration is to be replaced.

Radiographs

New patients with existing restorations and/or signs of periodontitis should have full mouth periapical radiographs taken routinely, unless contra-indicated for medical reasons. These radiographs should be taken with the long cone technique, as more details can be obtained than using short cones. Panoral radiographs are inadequate for periodontal or occlusal diagnosis. The following should be noted: width of the periodontal ligament, presence of worn teeth and closeness of occlusal surface to the roof of the pulp chamber, sclerosis of bone and hypercementosis, apical resorption or root fractures.

According to some authors it may be necessary to take standardised TMJ radiographs.[10]

Conclusions

The method of examination described can be performed by the experienced clinician in approximately 10 minutes, excluding the taking of radiographs. The examination will enable him to decide whether or not it is necessary to mount study casts on an articulator in order to glean further information. All patients requiring crowns, bridges or dentures—or with a history of migration of teeth—should have study casts made at the initial visit, and Chapter 2 will describe their construction, together with a more specific examination of the occlusion.

References

1 Berry D C, Poole D F G. Attrition: possible mechanisms of compensation. *J Oral Rehabil* 1976; **3**: 201–206.
2 Murphy T. Compensatory mechanisms in facial height adjustment to functional tooth attrition. *Aust Dent J* 1959; **4**: 312–323.
3 Williamson E H, Woelfel J B, Williams B H. A longitudinal study of rest position and centric occlusion. *Angle Orthod* 1975; **45**: 130–136.
4 Dawson P E. *Evaluation, diagnosis and treatment of occlusal problems*, p 102. St Louis: C V Mosby, 1974.
5 De Boever J. Functional disturbances of the temporomandibular joint, In *Temporomandibular joint function and dysfunction*, Edit Zarb G A, Carlsson G E, pp 197–201. Copenhagen: Munksgaard, 1979.
6 Setchell, D J. Personal communication, 1976.
7 Rugh J D, Solberg W K. Psychological implications in temporomandibular pain and dysfunction. In *Temporomandibular joint function and dysfunction*. Edit Zarb G A, Carlsson G E, p 249. Copenhagen: Munksgaard, 1979.
8 Johnstone D R, Templeton M. The feasibility of palpating the lateral pterygoid muscle. *J. Prosthet Dent* 1980; **44**: 318–323.
9 Schluger S, Yuodelis R A, Page R C. *Periodontal disease, basic phenomena, clinical management and occlusal and restorative inter-relationships*, p 311. Philadelphia: Lea and Febiger, 1977.
10 Weinberg L A. Clinical report on the aetiology and diagnosis of T M J dysfunction pain syndrome. *J Prosthet Dent,* 1980; **44**: 642–653.

Periodontal probe: Marquis Co, 15370 H Smith Road, Aurora, Colorado 80011, USA.

Occlusal articulating paper: Cottrells thin blue, Cottrell and Company, 15–17 Charlotte Street, London.

Occlusal tape: GHM Occlusion—PRÜF–FOLIE, 22 mm Hanel Medizinal Nurtingen; Precious Metals, 43 Devonshire Street, London W1, and Orthomax Dental Ltd, Carr House, Carr Bottom Road, Bradford BD5 9BJ.

Plastic foil: Artus Corporation, Box 511, Englewood, NJ 07631, USA; Precious Metals, 43 Devonshire Street, London W1, and Cottrell and Company, 15–17 Charlotte Street, London W1.

2 Examination of the Occlusion and Fabrication of Study Casts

This chapter will discuss the specific examination of the occlusion, the making of study casts and special examination methods such as diagnostic waxing and pantographic surveys.

Examination of the occlusion should follow the history taking and general examination described in Chapter 1. Although it is implied that tooth relationships will be observed, it is imperative that the position of the mandible relative to the maxilla is also considered. The clinical significance of the observations will be considered in Chapter 4.

Occlusal relationships

The following should be observed: the intercuspal position, the retruded contact position, the movement between the retruded contact position and intercuspal position, slide in occlusion, lateral contact positions and excursions, protrusive contact positions and excursions and the rest position.

It is important for the practitioner to know where to look and what to look for.

The intercuspal position (ICP)

This is the relationship of the mandible to the maxilla when the teeth are meshed maximally together (fig. 2.1).

Location The patient is asked to bring his teeth together in the position of best fit.

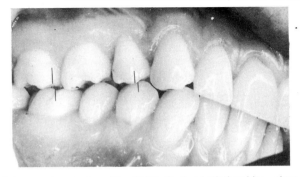

Fig. 2.1 The intercuspal contact position (ICP). Occlusal relationships—the teeth are in the position of best fit.

Observation   The overall arch relationships are noted, recording details of such irregularities as cross-bite and overerupted teeth. Horizontal overjet and overbite should be measured and recorded, especially noting if the upper and lower incisors and canines contact.

The retruded contact position (RCP)

The relationship of the mandible to the maxilla in which initial occlusion contact has occurred following closure about the posterior and most superior rotatory axis of the mandible (fig. 2.2).

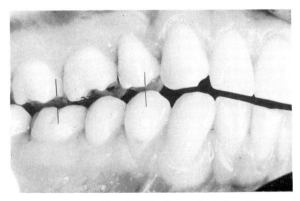

Fig. 2.2 The retruded contact position (RCP). Occlusal relationships—tooth contact has occurred following gentle guidance by the dentist so as to position the mandible more posteriorly than in figure 2.1. Note position of vertical lines compared to figure 2.1.

Location   Many techniques have been described for this procedure, but the most useful is that described by Dawson.[1] However slight modifications to Dawson's technique may be necessary to suit individual needs. Patients differ in the relative ease of location of this position and the technique for three stages of difficulty will be described.

Technique for 'easy' patient

The patient is placed in a reclining position in the dental chair and made as relaxed as possible. The head is cradled between the operator's chest and arm to offer stability. The patient should be spoken to calmly and confidently. The thumbs are placed on the chin, and the fingers support the body of the mandible as in figure 2.3. With slight downward pressure from the thumbs, and upward pressure from the fingers, the mandible is gently manipulated with oscillatory movements to a position just short of occlusal contacts. When the patient is felt to be relaxed, closure is then continued until initial contact is felt by the patient and he is asked to identify the area of such contact. The commonly used method of shaking the mandible violently does nothing more than precipitate fear in the patient and a tightening of the muscles which is contrary to what is required.

Patients who present slight difficulty in manipulation to RCP

The application of the 'tongue spatula technique' is sometimes used. The

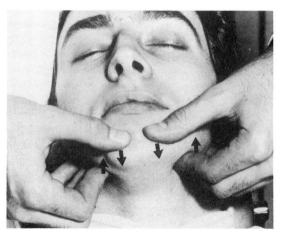

Fig. 2.3 Technique for locating the RCP for an 'easy patient'; see text for description. The thumbs press gently down on the chin, while the fingers support the body of the mandible. Oscillate the mandible up and down.

tongue spatula is placed between the upper and lower teeth as in figure 2.4 and the patient asked to contact it with the lower incisors. He maintains this position for approximately 5 min, so as to 'break up' proprioceptive reflexes and allow the muscles to 'forget' the habitual position of the mandible. The mandible can then be manipulated as described previously, to open and close against the tongue spatula which is then slowly removed and the patient's jaw closed to initial contact as before.

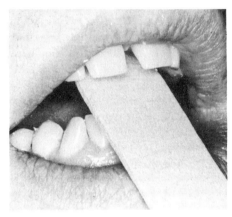

Fig. 2.4 Technique for locating the RCP for a patient with 'slight difficulty in manipulation'. The tongue spatula has been in position for 5 min to 'break up' proprioception. The chairside assistant slowly removes the spatula while the mandible is manipulated as before.

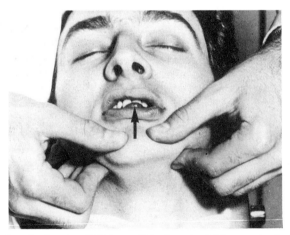

Fig. 2.5 Technique for locating RCP for a 'difficult patient'. The anterior jig (*arrowed*) has been in place for 15 min and the mandible is now being manipulated.

Patients who present more difficulty in manipulation

It may be necessary to fabricate an anterior jig, the function of which is to break up the proprioceptive reflex[2] (fig. 2.5).

The equipment needed is: autopolymerising acrylic such as Red Duralay, petroleum jelly, straight handpiece, tungsten-carbide trimmer, blue articulating paper.

The technique for making a jig is as follows:

(1) Apply petroleum jelly to the upper anterior teeth and block out any anterior diastemata.

(2) Mix autopolymerising resin.

(3) At the dough stage, the resin should be applied to the anterior teeth (fig. 2.6(a)) and shaped into a platform covering the palatal surfaces (fig. 2.6(b)) and extending about 3 mm over the incisal edge onto the labial surfaces. (fig. 2.6(c)).

(4) While the resin is soft guide the mandible as closely as possible to the retruded position, making sure that the lower incisors contact the palatal platform, and that there is sufficient material to allow posterior tooth separation of approximately 2 mm.

(5) As the resin begins to set, prise it off gently to prevent locking into undercuts and an excessive build-up of polymerisation heat.

(6) After it has set, replace the jig in the mouth and ensure that it is rigidly retained on the anterior teeth; if not, add more material to the fitting surface and repeat until rigidly retained.

(7) Place blue articulating paper on the jig and guide the mandible along left and right lateral paths (fig. 2.6(d)).

(8) Remove the jig and look at the markings and identify the movements of a single lower incisor against the upper platform (fig. 2.6(e)).

(9) Because of the direction of movement of the mandible (fig 2.6(f)) a lower incisor will trace V-shaped marks with the apex pointing palatally. Be aware that sometimes more than one tooth marks. Identify the mark from one incisor and remove the others.

(10) Trim the limbs of the V and repeat marking until the apex becomes smooth.

(11) Trim off limbs of the V leaving only the apex (fig. 2.6(g)).

(12) Replace in mouth and guide patient to contact this point.

(13) Leave in patient's mouth for approximately 10 minutes and then check for freedom of movement of the mandible (opening and closing). Guide the mandible and let the patient tap against the jig, and when free movement occurs remove the jig and locate the initial contacts.

Sometimes it may be necessary to have the jig in place for half an hour

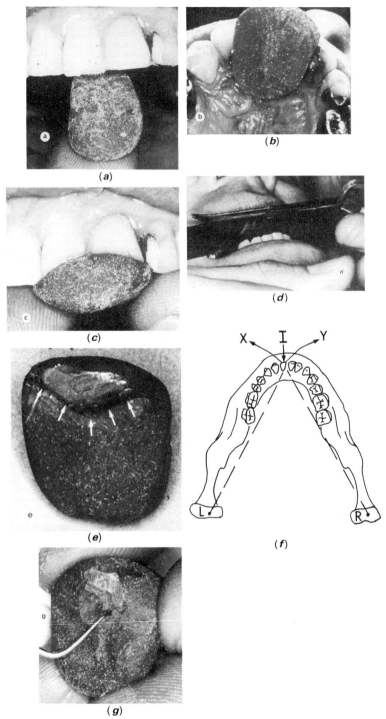

(a)

(b)

(c)

(d)

(e)

(f)

(g)

Fig. 2.6 Stages in the fabrication of an anterior jig. See the text for description. (**a**) Application of acrylic at dough stage. (**b**) Forming the palatal platform. (**c**) Labial coverage. (**d**) Blue articulating paper in place. (**e**) Mark of a lower incisor (*arrowed*) (**f**) Occlusal diagram of mandible to explain the reason for the V-shaped mark. L—left condyle, R—right condyle, I—lower incisor, LI—radius from L, RI—radius from R, IX—movement of lower incisor with left lateral excursion, IY—movement of lower incisor with right lateral excursion. Note: IX, IY form 'V' shape with I at the apex. (**g**) Limbs of V trimmed off.

prior to the examination and the patient may do this in the waiting room.

It may be necessary to make some form of disocclusion appliance (fig 2.7) which is adjusted periodically until the mandible can be manipulated easily. The fabrication will be described in Chapter 5 (occlusal splint).

Location with occlusal indicating tape

The procedure is as follows:

Specific location of the occlusal contacts can be obtained by the use of occlusal indicating tape.

(1) Dry the teeth with a gauze square.

(2) Place blue occlusal paper between the upper and lower teeth and direct the patient to rub his teeth in all directions.

(3) Instruct the patient to open.

(4) The chairside assistant places double-sided black occlusal tape between the upper and lower teeth, holding the tape in Miller's forceps as in figure 2.8.

(5) Manipulate the mandible to the retruded position, and instruct the patient to tap once in this position.

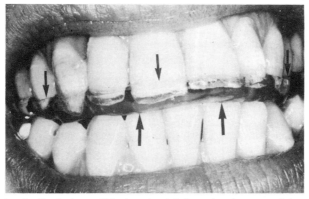

Fig. 2.7 Occlusal splint for 'very difficult patient'. Adjusted and worn until the mandible can be manipulated easily (see Chapter 5 for fabrication)

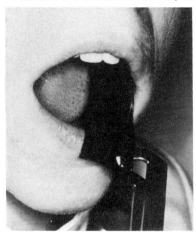

Fig. 2.8 Insertion of occlusal tape held in forceps by the chairside assistant.

(6) Remove the tape, warm a mouth mirror and observe the black marks on the blue background. It must be emphasised that it is impossible to locate occlusal contacts precisely with the blue articulating paper alone, owing to its thickness.[3] The blue layer merely aids the subsequent marking with the thin occlusal tape and is not always necessary.

Observation   Note: teeth in contact, area of contact, horizontal and vertical overjet and ease of manipulation.

Movement from RCP to ICP

Location   Manipulate the mandible to the RCP and then instruct the patient to 'squeeze' the teeth together until a position of 'best fit' is reached. Repeat the procedure using occlusal tapes as follows:
(1) Teeth dried
(2) Blue tape and teeth rubbed in all directions.
(3) Mouth open and dryness of teeth obtained by assistant using suction.
(4) Insert red occlusal tape. (Double-sided red GHM tape is not available. Cut a strip of single-sided tape, twice the length of the forceps beaks, fold it back on itself and secure in the forceps. Ensure that the dull sides are facing outwards.)
(5) Manipulate to RCP and mark, then instruct the patient to squeeze teeth.

(6) Remove red tape.
(7) Insert black tape.
(8) Manipulate to RCP and tap teeth together once.
(9) Insert green tape.
(10) Tap once in ICP (fig. 2.9).

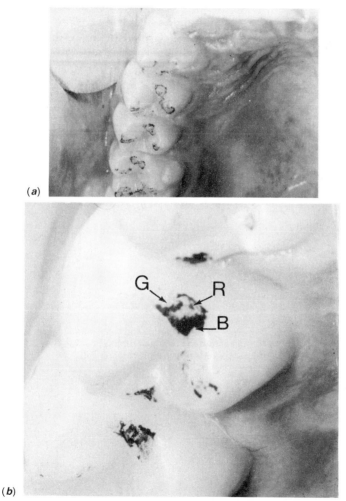

Fig. 2.9(a) The initial blue layer marking the teeth. This is 'gross' and does not represent true contacts. It is not always required. (*b*) Red (R)—slide from RCP to ICP; green (G)— ICP contact; black (B) – RCP contact.

Observation

At the incisors note the:

(1) Dimensions of slide from retruded to intercuspal positions.
(2) Direction—whether slide is straightforwards, forwards to one side or only to one side.
(3) Vertical and horizontal components of slide. This is the change in the distance between the upper and lower incisors in the vertical and horizontal planes occurring during the slide from RCP to ICP. Figures 2.10(*a*) and (*b*) show a large vertical component and a small horizontal component at the incisal region. Compare this with figures 2.11(*a*) and (*b*) which show a small vertical and a large horizontal component.

Note the contacting surfaces from the marks made by the occlusal tapes (fig. 2.10) the initial contact in the RCP (black), the surfaces in contact while the slide (if any) occurs (red) and ICP contacts (green).

(4) Ease of slide. Determine the degree of freedom of movement from RCP to ICP and whether this movement is influenced in any way by the inclined plane of the opposing cusps. In other words is the movement forced?

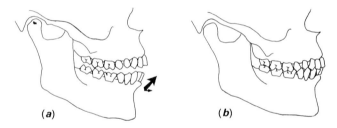

(*a*)   (*b*)

Fig. 2.10 Slide from (*a*) RCP to (*b*) ICP. Large vertical and small horizontal components.— RCP: the arrow in the incisal region shows the direction of movement to the ICP. Note that condylar movement is mainly rotation.

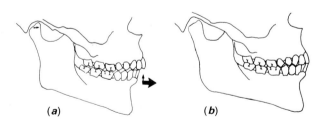

(*a*)   (*b*)

Fig. 2.11 Slide from (*a*) RCP to (*b*) ICP. Small vertical and large horizontal components. (*a*) Arrows in the incisor and condylar regions show the direction of movement to the ICP (*b*) Note that condylar movement is mainly translation.

Lateral positions and excursions

Locations and observations are made on both the working side and the non-working side.

Working side contacts

Contacts of teeth made on the side of the occlusion towards which the mandible has been moved[4] (fig. 2.12).

Location   The patient is instructed to close into the ICP and then move to whichever side is to be investigated. Frequently, the patient may have difficulty in moving to the required side. This may be facilitated by the patient using a face mirror to observe the movement of the lower jaw. Instruct the patient to move to the edge-to-edge position, and slightly beyond (the cross-over position). Ideally the contact should be located from the RCP as well but this is frequently difficult. Once located the contacting surfaces can be marked as before.

Observation   With the teeth in contact during lateral excursion, note whether:
(1) There is group function (contact of multiple teeth on the working side) (fig. 2.12(*a*)) or
(2) There is canine guidance (contact only between the canines with the other teeth separated or discluded) (fig. 2.12(*b*)). Frequently, there will be a combination of (1) and (2) such that initially there is group function, but in the edge to edge position only the canines contact.
(3) The guiding teeth move excessively.
(4) The lateral movement is smooth or restricted.
(5) The teeth are in contact in the cross-over position.

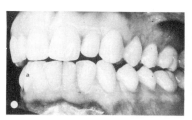 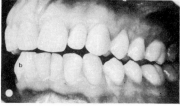

Fig. 2.12 Left lateral excursion. (*left*) Group function: multiple teeth contact on the working side. (*right*) With further excursion this becomes canine guidance—only the canines contact.

Non-working side contacts (balancing side contacts)

Contacts of teeth made on the side of the occlusion from which the mandible moves during lateral excursion, that is the side opposite the working side. For example, right lateral excursion, working side—right; non-working side—left.

Location   The location non-working side contacts can be made at the same time as the working side contacts. However, the operator should support the mandible on the non-working side while doing this (fig. 2.13) as there is a tendency for the patient to skirt around the non-working side contacts.

Observation   Note:
(1) Presence or absence of non-working side contacts.
(2) Movement of teeth on the non-working side.
(3) Corresponding working side contacts.

Protrusive positions and excursions

There are two relationships: straight protrusion, or lateral protrusion, that is movement forward and slightly to one side.

Location   Instruct the patient to close into the ICP and then slide forward until the incisors come edge-to-edge. Again, the face mirror simplifies this

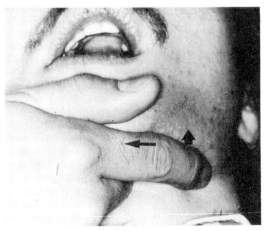

Fig. 2.13 Right lateral excursion. Supporting the mandible on the left, non-working side contacts are observed on the patient's left side.

procedure. Similarly, for lateral protrusion instruct the patient to close to the ICP then move forward and to one side. Specific contacts may be located with tapes.

Observation   Note:
(1) The direction of movements.
(2) The mobility of teeth during jaw movements.
(3) Whether the teeth are in contact during movement.
(4) The presence or absence of posterior contact during protrusive movements.

The rest position

The relationship of the mandible to the maxilla when the patient is relaxed and sitting upright.

Location   Position the patient comfortably and upright in the chair. Use one of the many prosthetic methods to assess interocclusal clearance. For example, tell the patient to lick the lips and swallow, say 'Mmm . . .' relax, then part the lips and assess the space between 1|1 and 1|1.

Observation   Interocclusal clearance is observed. However, be aware that many factors can influence the rest position such as stress, pain, and muscle hyperactivity.

Special investigations

Study casts
Study casts provide an essential record of the dentition and it is important that these casts are carefully fabricated. Compare figure 2.14(*a*) with figure 2.14(*b*) and note the discrepancy between the occlusal surfaces owing to distortion of the alginate impressions caused in this case by carelessly allowing excess alginate at the heels of the tray to contact the worktops while the stone was setting in the impression.

Equipment required: either reversible hydrocolloid or irreversible hydrocolloid (alginate), 'Rimlock tray'[11] (conventional perforated tray is adequate), 2 × 2 inch gauze square, rubber bowl and spatula.

The teeth should be cleaned and the correct sized trays selected. The occlusal surfaces are lightly wiped with a gauze while the chairside assistant

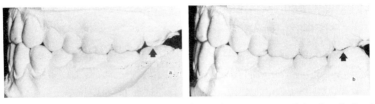

Fig. 2.14 Distorted study casts resulting from the unsupported heels of the lower impression resting on the bench. (*left*) Distorted casts ($\overline{8}$ is out of occlusion). (*right*) Correct cast.

mixes the impression material according to the manufacturer's instructions. A small amount of alginate is taken on the finger and applied to the occlusal surfaces of the teeth, forcing it into the grooves (fig. 2.15). (With reversible hydrocolloid, syringe material may be used.) It is important that saliva does not contaminate the surface of this layer, as it may affect the uniform setting of the whole impression. The loaded tray is inserted. The impression is removed when set and covered with the damp gauze or placed in a humidor prior to pouring. Ensure that any unsupported heels of the impression material are not left resting on the worktop, otherwise this will cause distortion of the impression. The cast should be poured with minimal delay and based. It should have a date and be stored for future reference. (It is frequently useful to make a second model for diagnostic 'cutting' and waxing of teeth.)

Use of study casts

(1) *For future reference*   It may not be possible to make a definitive

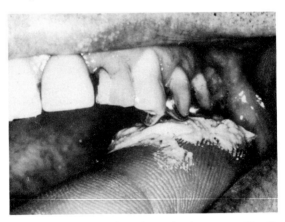

Fig. 2.15 Forcing alginate into the occlusal grooves with a finger.

diagnosis without study casts. Referral to the original casts enables the operator to determine the presence or absence of occlusal deterioration with time.

(2) *Tooth positions and surface features*   It is frequently easier to locate diastemata, fractured cusps, and worn areas, on study casts than directly in the mouth.

(3) *Intercuspal relationships*   The cast may be held manually in the intercuspal position to observe tooth relationships.

(4) *Mounting of casts*   Casts mounted in a semi-adjustable articulator (fig. 2.16) will facilitate evaluation of tooth relationships in the various jaw positions, that is retruded contact position, intercuspal position, protrusive and lateral positions. The procedures for carrying out such mounting will be described in Chapter 5.

(5) *Diagnostic waxing*   Some cases require a diagnostic waxing or tooth repositioning (fig. 2.17) before a treatment plan can be evolved. Either a single tooth or a whole dentition may be waxed up. It is a pity that this procedure is often dismissed as a waste of time since it provides much valuable information regarding aesthetics, contour, potential preparations, the occlusal plane, the need for elective periodontal surgery to increase crown height and the need for orthodontic treatment. It also provides a template for the fabrication of temporary restorations.

Pantographic survey

A dental pantograph is a device used to trace mandibular movement and

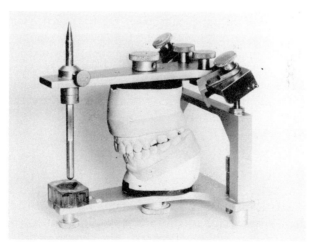

Fig. 2.16 Study casts mounted in a semi-adjustable articulator (Whip Mix).

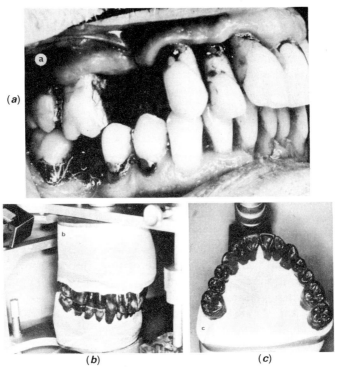

(*a*)

(*b*)   (*c*)

2.17(*a*) Clinical picture (*b*) and (*c*) Diagnostic waxing.

consists essentially of an upper and lower facebow each attached to the corresponding dental arch (fig. 2.18). Styli attached to one bow contact a flat plate on the opposite bow. As the patient performs lateral jaw movements, the styli will trace their paths on the plates. Some authors[5] consider that the non-reproducibility of pantographic tracings provides valuable graphic information regarding the need for occlusal therapy prior to extensive restorative dentistry.

Conclusions

This article has described the procedures used to locate and observe the various occlusal relationships. The advantages of study casts have been outlined, and the pantograph briefly mentioned. In Chapter 5 mounting of the casts in articulators will be described. The clinical significance of the observations will be described in Chapters 3 and 4.

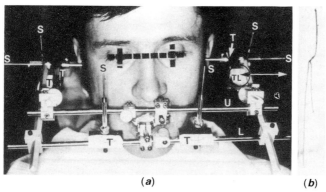

(*a*)   (*b*)

Fig. 2.18 Pantograph (from the Stuart system). (*a*) Assembled on patient. Upper bow—U; lower bow—L; styli—S; tracing plates—T. (Left horizontal plate—TL.) (*b*) Enlargement of the tracings from the left horizontal tracing plate.

References

1 Dawson P E. *Evaluation, diagnosis and treatment of occlusal problems*, p 56. St Louis. C V Mosby 1974.

2 Lucia V O. A technique for recording centric relation. *J. Prosthet Dent* 1964; **14**: 492–505.

3 Kelleher M G D. A laboratory investigation of marking materials used for the detection of occlusal contact. MSc Thesis, University of London, 1978.

4 Glossary of prosthodontic terms. *J. Prosthet Dent* 1977; **38**: 70–109.

5 Crispin B J, Myers G E, Clayton J A. Effects of occlusal therapy on pantographic reproducibility of mandibular border movements. *J. Prosthet Dent* 1978; **40**: 29–34.

Red Duralay: Duralay Inlay Pattern Resin—Reliance Dental Mfg Co, Worth, Ill, USA 60482 and Cottrell & Co.

Tungsten carbide trimmer: Jotta Burr No 146/22—Cottrell & Co, 15–17 Charlotte Street, London W1.

Blue occlusal paper: Cottrell & Co, 15–17 Charlotte Street, London W1. Thin blue.

Black occlusal tape: GHM Occlusion—PRÜF–FOLIE, 22 mm Hanzel Medizinal Nurtingen, Precious Metals, 43 Devonshire Street, London W1, and Cottrell and Company, 15–17 Charlotte Street, London W1.

Rimlock tray: Caulk Company Rimlock Tray—M J Dental Supplies Ltd, 100 High Street, Ramsey, Camb PE17 1BS.

---

3 The Clinical Significance of the Examination Findings

A step by step procedure for examining an occlusion was described in Chapters 1 and 2, the clinical significance of the findings will now be discussed in the same sequence.

This Chapter should be used in conjunction with Chapters 1 and 2 to help the practitioner determine which cases require a more thorough analysis of the occlusion, and to assist him in developing a plan of treatment.

The clinical significance of the findings of the examination will be influenced by:

(1) The extent of restorative therapy required.
(2) The age of the patient. The 22-year-old with advanced wear and large restorations requires a different approach to the 65-year-old also exhibiting advanced wear.
(3) The experience of the dentist.
(4) The competence of the technical assistance.

It is pointless to carry out occlusal therapy if this is to be followed by provision of restorations incorporating greater discrepancies than were originally present. The profession has been sadly lacking in its co-operation with and training of dental technicians. The current trend towards technicians being remote from the surgery with communication often being poorly carried out on 'bits of paper' or the prescription being left to the technician, is one to be discouraged. It is imperative that the profession educates itself and the technicians to produce the many simple restorations that are required in a manner which is not damaging to the dentition.

History

Complaint

The nature of the patient's original complaint may give the dentist a guide as to how extensive his occlusal examination should be:

(1) No complaint: routine examination; occlusal examination will be minimal.

(2) Pain in the face, with tenderness in the regions of the muscles of mastication and temporomandibular joints, clicking of the joints during jaw movement and limitation of mandibular movement are indicative of TMJ dysfunction and should be a warning not to embark on extensive restorative therapy until remission from the dysfunction has been achieved. Extensive alteration of the occlusion by way of restorations at this stage may exacerbate the symptoms and make it difficult to achieve comfort.

(3) Toothache precipitated by chewing, as well as hot and cold stimuli, may indicate a split tooth, often caused by a faulty occlusion.[1]

(4) The patient who requests and requires extensive restorative therapy must have a thorough occlusal examination.

Response to questions

(1) TMJ dysfunction symptoms   As for (2) above.

(2) *Bruxism*   A history of bruxism, coupled with that of fractured or uncemented restorations (fig. 3.1), fractured drifting or severely worn teeth, calls for a more thorough occlusal investigation. Where restorations

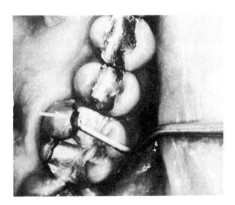

Fig. 3.1 Fracture of the palatal cusp of |6, in a patient with large amalgams and a history of bruxism. The patient reported that the fracture occurred while grinding his teeth in a traffic jam.

have failed mechanically, the dentist must make some positive decisions about the occlusal prescriptions for replacements.

(3) *Oral habits* such as pencil or lip sucking are significant for two reasons: drifting anterior teeth may be due to the habit and not the occlusion or periodontitis (Chapter 2); cessation of the habit may allow simple realignment (fig. 3.2). Secondly, the habit may have developed in order to prevent cross clashing of cusps due to large occlusal interferences.[2]

(4) *Looseness of teeth* The patient's subjective impression of tooth mobility is important, and will be discussed later (see clinical significance of mobility).

(5) *Drifting of teeth*, particularly the upper anterior segment—may indicate:

(i) Advancing periodontitis.

(ii) Oral habits, such as pencil biting.

(iii) Posterior deflective contact, that is, an occlusal contact that deviates the mandible from its original path of closure into another path; causing an anterior adaptive mandibular path of closure, resulting in the lower anterior teeth pushing the upper anteriors labially (figs 3.3(*a*) and (*b*)).

(iv) Loss of posterior occlusal support.

(v) Change of elasticity of circumoral musculature with ageing, altering the muscle equilibrium.

(vi) Altered anterior crown contour, typically associated with overcontoured bonded porcelain restorations.

A history of drifting of the upper anterior teeth requires careful examination of the periodontium and posterior occlusion. However the position of a

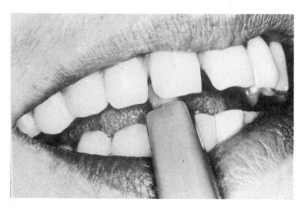

Fig. 3.2 Habit pushing 1| labially (Courtesy Mr V. J. Ward).

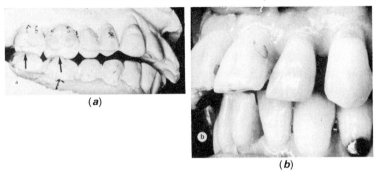

(a)

(b)

Fig. 3.3 Posterior deflective contacts causing an anterior adaptive path of closure and labial movement of the upper anterior segment. (*a*) RCP right side—contact between 76| and |76. (*b*) ICP left side 'adaptive' position. Lower incisors contact the uppers which have moved labially. There is no pocketing (see fig. 1.3).

drifted tooth may be stable and acceptable to the patient. Not all such teeth should be realigned. Periodontitis, if present, must be treated and good study casts made for future reference.

(6) *Pain in the teeth*   All the obvious and common causes of dental pain must be eliminated. However, pain on biting, immediately following placement of a restoration may indicate a high spot which should be investigated and tested by adjustment; or pain to hot and cold and chewing suggests a split tooth (fig. 3.4), often in premolars with MOD restorations, particularly if such teeth have non-working side interferences or initial contacts in the retruded contact position. The diagnosis may require confirmation by:

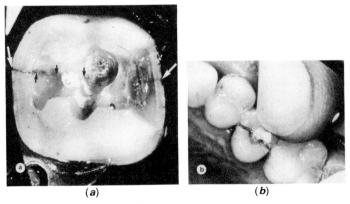

(a)   (b)

Fig. 3.4 Tooth fracture. (*a*) Mesiodistal fracture present beneath an old amalgam (black background is rubber dam). (*b*) Separating cusps to reveal a mesiodistal fracture.

- Adjusting the occlusion on the tooth.
- Radiographs to ensure no periapical abnormality.
- Vitality testing.
- Gently spreading apart the buccal and lingual cusps with the fingertips and noting any painful response. Obvious complete fractures will separate at this time (fig. 3.4).
- Removal of the restoration, preferably after isolation with rubber dam to investigate the pulpal floor directly.
- Transillumination with a fibre-optic light source.

(7) *Mechanical restorative failures* always require careful occlusal examination to determine the cause of such failures which could be: poor tooth preparation or manipulation of restorative materials, and/or detrimental occlusal factors.

Extra-oral examination

Temporomandibular joint
Irregular and limited movement coupled with muscle symptoms indicate TMJ dysfunction. It is foolhardy to embark on extensive definitive restorations, until the dysfunction symptoms have been relieved. For management of this condition, the reader is referred to Zarb and Speck.[3]

Clicking of the joint There is no evidence to suppose that this can be relieved by management of the occlusion.

In the author's opinion, the general practitioner should confine his occlusal efforts to the provision of a sound restorative service and not become involved in the controversial subject of its role in the relief of TMJ pain. However, as stated previously, when restorations are required careful occlusal management is necessary to prevent an exacerbation of symptoms.

Muscles of mastication
Severe sensitivity to palpation should warn the practitioner against carrying out extensive restorations involving occlusal surfaces until such sensitivity has subsided, either as a result of therapy or spontaneously in the natural cycle of such conditions.

Intra-oral examination

Muscles
Sensitivity in the region of the lateral pterygoid muscles is particularly significant.[4]

It should be noted that the two heads of this pterygoid muscle are inserted into the region of the joint (fig. 3.5). Grant[5] considers that the superior head functions 'to oppose the condyle and the articular eminence', within a small range of opening, beyond which Storey considers[6] that it serves to move the disc downwards and forwards as the inferior head pulls the mandible in the same direction. Following excursive movements of the mandible, either in bruxism or mastication, contractions of the elevator muscles of mastication will tend to reseat the condyle in the fossa, while its backward movement is controlled by relaxation of the contracted lateral pterygoid muscles.

Mandibular excursions to the left involve contraction of the right lateral pterygoid and vice versa. Bruxism will be associated with alternate contraction and relaxation of this muscle. Krough-Poulson and Olsson consider[7] that faceting associated with bruxism should be coupled with the findings of the muscle examination. For example, whenever muscle sensitivity can be associated with the faceting and the teeth to be restored are the ones exhibiting the faceting, it is prudent to adjust the occlusion on these teeth

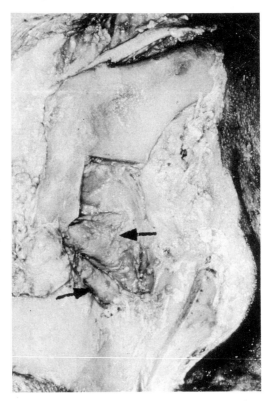

Fig. 3.5 The coronoid process and part of the ramus have been removed to reveal the two portions of the lateral pterygoid muscle (*arrowed*). Contraction of the lateral pterygoid muscle moves the condyle forward while maintaining apposition of the condyle, disc and eminentia. (Courtesy of Mr B. J. Parkins.)

prior to tooth preparation (provided that the faceted area would be cut in tooth preparation) and assess the patient's response, since preparation for restoration would itself eliminate the occlusal contacts. It is advisable to eliminate these contacts and be certain that the patient is comfortable before the tooth is prepared, otherwise many hours of 'grinding in' can result (figs. 3.6(*a*), (*b*) and (*c*)).

Extensive restorations should not be carried out in the presence of severe muscle sensitivity in any of the masticatory muscles.

Teeth and periodontium

Both groups A ('wear' patients) and B (periodontitis-susceptible patients) will require plaque control and motivation prior to restorative therapy. However, the 'wear' patient will require more thorough initial examination of the occlusion, since it is likely that restorative therapy would be commenced fairly early. Furthermore, these patients are likely to encounter problems of differential wear of materials, and hence the occlusal surfaces of restorations should be carefully prescribed at an early stage.

The periodontitis patient, however, usually requires a prolonged phase of plaque control and motivation and assessment of tissue response, with only simple restorative therapy in the early stages. For these patients a more detailed evaluation of the occlusion can usually be left until a later stage. The belief that mechanical therapy will cure the periodontitis is to be discouraged. There is a danger that the early mounting of study casts and use of articulators, could suggest to the patient that their problems could be solved simply by 'carpentry'.

The patient with advanced periodontitis and missing teeth for whom early extractions are deemed necessary, may need mounting of study casts at an early stage, but management of these cases is not considered to be within the scope of this chapter.

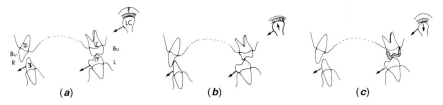

(*a*)   **(*b*)**   **(*c*)**

Fig. 3.6 Frontal view at three levels showing 3| 3| and |7 |7 and the left condyle (LC) and fossa (F) relationships. L—patient's left; R—patient's right; Bu—buccal. (*a*) In right lateral excursion the guidance is primarily from |7 palatal cusp against |7 buccal cusp (non-working side contacts). The left condyle is not seated in the fossa due to the cuspal contacts, but since adaptation has occurred over many years the patient is relatively comfortable. (*b*) |7 prepared for a crown. In the right lateral excursion 3| |3 now contact and muscle contraction moves the left condyle higher into the fossa. A temporary crown is placed. (*c*) New crown positioned on |7 (shaded). The shape of the palatal cusp differs from that in (*a*). During a right lateral excursion the left condyle is again moved inferiorly. Frequently the patient will complain that |7 is high and the dentist starts to grind it only to go through the crown or break the porcelain on a bonded crown. The net result is usually to blame the technician whereas the fault was the dentist's.

Teeth present/teeth absent

Not all missing teeth require replacement and the occlusal indications for replacement of missing units are:
(1) Loss of posterior support affecting the anterior teeth causing drifting, increasing mobility or wear (fig. 3.7).
(2) Impairment of function.
(3) Instability caused by movement of isolated teeth.

Pocket depth and mobility

These should be considered together. The common causes of excessive tooth mobility are:
(1) Periodontitis (fig. 3.8). Note the presence of bleeding, pocketing and alveolar bone loss.
(2) Occlusal forces. Excessive occlusal forces, may be direct, when the opposing teeth are deflective or bruxing contacts (fig. 3.9), or after periodontal treatment, when the treated tooth will have a healthy periodontium, but since it is reduced in quantity due to the disease it may now exhibit increased mobility under normal occlusal loads (see fig. 3.13). Alternatively, the forces may originate indirectly, when a posterior deflective contact leads to an anterior path of closure causing a distant tooth to be traumatised (fig. 3.9); or a posterior tooth is the favourite site for bruxing, but bruxism on this tooth may affect a distant tooth, resulting in the latter becoming mobile (fig. 3.10).

Other causes of altered mobility which should be noted for differential diagnosis are:

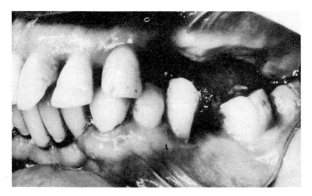

Fig. 3.7 Loss of posterior support has resulted in labial movement of |123. Occlusal support is required.

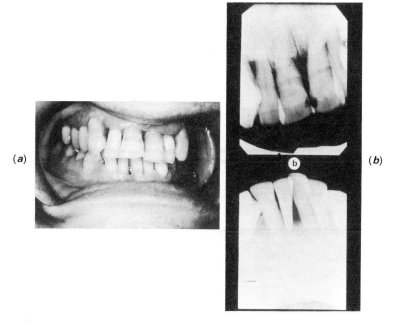

Fig. 3.8 The patient had complained of increasing mobility of 21|12 and drifting of 1|. The dentist having recently been on an occlusion course noticed occlusal deflective contacts and referred the patient for an occlusal adjustment, but note (**a**) the inflammation and (**b**) bone loss. The mobility was due to periodontitis.

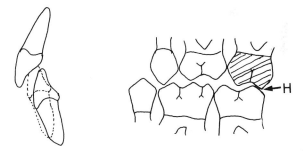

Fig. 3.9 Sagittal view. High crown on the |7. H—high spot. Possibilities: (1) The patient complains and the crown is ground, (2) |7 and/or |7 become mobile, and/or (3) |7 and/or |7 wear or break, and/or (4) the mandible adopts a new path of closure to avoid the high spots. The upper incisors are now traumatised by the lowers (*dotted outline*) and become mobile, move, wear or fracture.

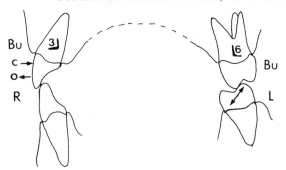

Fig. 3.10 Frontal view showing 3| 3| and |6 [6. L—patient's left; R—patient's right; Bu— buccal. Bruxing on |6 [6 results in contact between 3| 3| which can become mobile, move, wear or fracture. C—effect of the circumoral muscles; O—the effect of occlusal forces.

- Diurnal variation. Teeth free from periodontal disturbance normally exhibit slight mobility, which has been shown to vary throughout the day.
- Periapical inflammation.
- External trauma, for example a blow to the face.
- Pregnancy.
- Fractured roots.
- Shortened roots owing to overzealous orthodontic therapy (fig. 3.11) or apicectomy.
- Congenitally short or tapered roots.
- Neoplasms.

In order to assess the significance of mobility the following information is required. Is the patient aware of the mobility and if so does it concern him? Are the teeth stable?

A tooth can be mobile with no subsequent change (no increasing or decreasing mobility). A tooth can be mobile, and the mobility increasing at each assessment period. Finally, a tooth can be mobile, the mobility increasing over a period of time but becoming stable, at an increased level.

These classifications are important in terms of therapy and imply that a charting system for reassessment is essential.

The clinical significance of mobility
Remember that mobility is a symptom or sign not a disease.

Increasing mobility about which the patient is concerned
(1) In the presence of pocketing—very common and often associated with

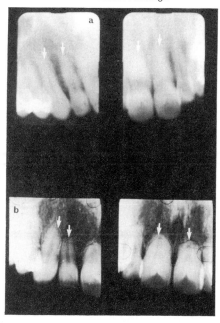

Fig. 3.11 Reduced support due to root shortening. (*upper*) Radiographs before treatment (poor quality since these were copies of the dentist's originals). (*lower*) 4 years later following 2 years of orthodontic treatment. Note resorbed roots. (Courtesy of Mr J. Zamet)

bone loss, primarily the result of plaque induced inflammation (figs 3.8(*a*) and (*b*)). Occasionally, investigation of the occlusion and minor correction is required to initially reduce mobility to give patient comfort. However, therapy is directed to resolution of inflammation by plaque control and elimination of pocketing, if necessary.

Current research clearly demonstrates that plaque is the major aetiological factor, and to ignore this is to court failure. If increasing mobility remains following resolution of the inflammation see the paragraphs below.

(2) In the absence of pocketing or marginal inflammation mobility is usually due to trauma from occlusion and requires investigation and elimination of aetiologic factors. Figure 3.12(*a*) shows a patient with a mobile upper lateral incisor in the absence of inflammation or pocketing but showing a widened periodontal ligament radiographically (fig. 3.12(*c*)). The patient gave a history of bruxism and right lateral pterygoid sensitivity and figure 3.12(*b*) shows the most favoured bruxing position, with contact on the right molars but also on the lateral incisor. Figure 3.12(*d*) shows the radiograph three years after occlusal therapy: note the altered appearance

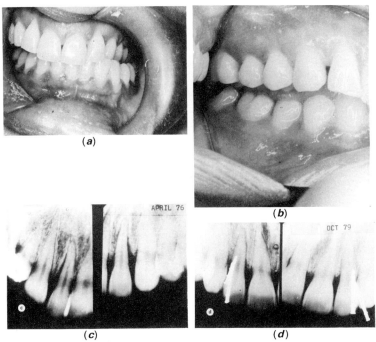

(a)

(b)

(c)   (d)

Fig. 3.12 Mobile 2|2 due to heavy occlusal forces. See text for details. (Compare with figure 3.10) (**a**) Patient's favourite bruxing position. Note absence of inflammation. (**b**) Non-working side contact 7| |7 corresponding to (**a**)–(**d**). Radiographs. (**d**) Radiographs 3 years following occlusal adjustment. (X-ray angulation is slightly different from (**c**), but radio-paque points depict base of crevice.)

of the periodontal ligament space. (It could be argued that altered angulation of the radiograph accounts for the change. However, the decreased mobility and clinical acceptability make this unlikely.) Extraction of this tooth (suggested by the patient's own dentist) was definitely contra-indicated since there was absence of pocketing and the bone loss associated with the root was not affecting the adjacent teeth which would be potential abutments. Placement of a bridge without correction of the occlusion would have resulted in mechanical failure of the bridge, because the bridge could have been subjected to the same forces as the natural tooth.

Increasing mobility of which the patient is unaware

(1) In the presence of pocketing or marginal inflammation this requires further investigation of the occlusion following plaque control and elimination of inflammation, assuming that the mobility continues to increase following these procedures.

(2) In the absence of pocketing or marginal inflammation this requires observation and further investigation and treatment of the occlusion if the mobility continues to increase.

Increased mobility of which the patient is unaware
In either the presence or absence of marginal inflammation or pocketing, usually should be noted and reassessed at subsequent recalls. Obviously inflammation and pocketing must be treated.

Increased mobility which concerns the patient following the correction of periodontitis
This requires further occlusal analysis and correction possibly in conjunction with splinting (fig. 3.13).

Increased mobility, of which the patient is unaware, remaining after correction of periodontitis
This requires occlusal analysis to assess whether simple adjustment can reduce this (to stabilise the occlusion and prevent food packing and drifting). However, the patient should not be subjected to time-consuming

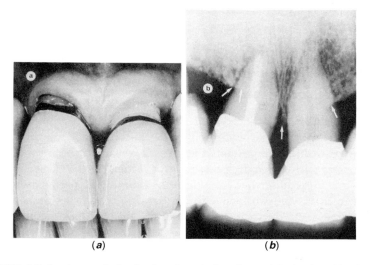

(a)   (b)

Fig. 3.13(a) Following surgical reduction of pocketing, the teeth had reduced but healthy periodontia. They were splinted to act as bridge abutments and because normal occlusal loads produced a degree of mobility which was unacceptable to the patient. (Note: the patient had a low lip line, so that the margins of the crowns were not exposed in function. Supragingival margins did not compromise the gingivae.) (**b**) The post-surgical bone levels are *arrowed*.

and expensive procedures, since these have not been demonstrated to be necessary.

However, basic guidelines should be tempered by clinical prudence. Consider the situation in which inflammation has been eliminated, there is residual increased mobility which does not concern the patient, and multiple crowns are required, for example for bridge abutments, or due to failed restorations. When the bone support is greatly reduced, the splinting of these 'necessary' crowns should be considered, since subsequent drifting, or increasing mobility, or increased mobility which concerns the patient could prove difficult to correct without replacing the crowns. If the crowns are joined, it is implied that the periodontium must not be compromised by overcontoured solder or cast joints.

Remember that in the presence of untreated periodontitis the splinting of teeth does not retard the progression of disease and that following elimination of periodontitis mobile teeth only require splinting to make them functionally acceptable to the patient or to prevent instability leading, for example, to drifting.

Fremitus
It is important to decide whether or not a tooth exhibiting fremitus is an initial contact on the retruded path of closure; or exhibits fremitus at the end of a slide, that is, a posterior deflective contact resulting in an anterior slide and precipitating anterior tooth fremitus.

In the first instance the involved tooth may require adjustment, whereas in the second it is the posterior tooth which would require adjustment.

Tooth crowns
Young patients with advanced wear, requiring multiple restorations should have a thorough analysis made of their occlusions, since the problems of differential wear are important. Faceting, non-working side contact, and lateral pterygoid sensitivity should be investigated and when all three factors are present further investigation is indicated particularly if the faceted teeth are non-working side contacts and require restoration.

Fractured teeth, microcracks, uncemented bridges and fractured restorations indicate the need for further investigation of the occlusion before providing new restorations (this will be referred to in Chapter 7).

Radiographs
(1) *Width of periodontal ligament*   The commonest cause of a widened periodontal ligament is periodontitis. Widening of the periodontal liga-

ment in the absence of pocketing but with increased mobility is a sign of trauma from occlusion.

(2) *Wear* The nearness of worn occlusal surfaces to the pulp is important when restorations are required as it may not be possible to remove sufficient tooth to provide room for the restorative material without exposing the pulp. Furthermore, the pulp may already be exposed through wear (figs 3.14(*a*) and (*b*)). The height of the adjacent bone must also be assessed, since reduction of the occlusal tissue for restoration may result in solder joints encroaching on the embrasures preventing good plaque control. It may also be necessary to carry out elective periodontal surgery in order to increase crown height before commencing restorations. If this is contemplated the level of the root furcation must be assessed lest it be exposed during surgery (figs 3.15(*a*)–(*d*)).

(3) *Sclerosis of bone and hypercementosis, apical resorption and root fractures* are all important if the teeth are to be extracted or are mobile and are to be used for bridge abutments.

Conclusion

The clinical significance of the findings of the general examination have been considered. Chapter 4 will continue with the significance of the findings related to occlusal relationships and special investigations.

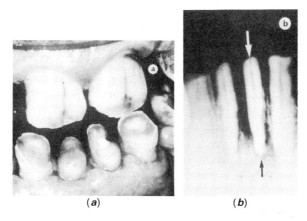

(*a*)   (*b*)

Fig. 3.14(*a*) Wear has resulted in the exposure of the pulp in ⌐1. (*b*) Radiographic appearance. Note exposure and periapical radiolucency.

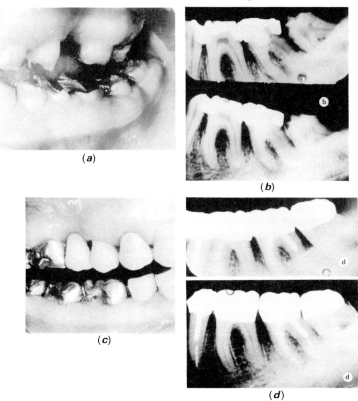

Fig. 3.15(a) and (b) Advanced wear. Note the height of the clinical crowns, the relationship to the pulp chamber, the relationship of the interdental bone to the crown length and the relationship of the furcation areas to crown length and bone. (c) and (d) Case following tissue resection (by Mr B. Keiser) root therapy (by Mr E. Nicholls) and restoration.

References

1 Silvestri A R, Singh I. Treatment rationale of fractured posterior teeth. *J Am Dent Assoc* 1978; **97**: 806–810.
2 Dawson P E. Evaluation and diagnosis and treatment of occlusal problems, pp 19, 295. St Louis: C V Mosby, 1974.
3 Zarb G A, Speck J E. The treatment of mandibular dysfunction, In: *Temporomandibular joint function and dysfunction*, Zarb G A, Carlsson G E (ed) p 373. Copenhagen: Munksgaard, 1979.
4 De Boever J A. Functional disturbances of the temporomandibular joint, In: *Temporomandibular joint function and dysfunction*, Zarb G A, Carlsson G E (ed) p 202. Copenhagen: Munksgaard, 1979.

5 Grant P G. Lateral pterygoid: two muscles? *Am J Anat* 1973; **138:** 1–9.
6 Storey A T. Controversies related to temporomandibular joint function and dysfunction. In: *Temporomandibular joint function and dysfunction*, Zarb G A, Carlsson G E (ed), p 435. St Louis: C V Mosby, 1979.
7 Krogh-Pousen W G, Olsson A. Management of the occlusion of the teeth, In *Facial pain and mandibular dysfunction*. Schwartz L, Chayes C M (ed), p 263–280. Philadelphia: W B Saunders, 1968.

4 Further Clinical Significance of the Examination Findings

In this chapter, the clinical significance of the findings of the specific occlusal examination will be considered in the same order as the examination procedures outlined in Chapter 2. It is assumed that for many cases study casts are mounted on a semi-adjustable articulator to enable the dentist to assess the occlusion further. Articulators will be considered in Chapter 5.

Occlusal relationships

The sequence for the examination was: (1) the intercuspal position (ICP), (2) the retruded contact position (RCP), (3) the slide from the retruded contact position to the intercuspal position, (4) lateral contact positions and excursions, (5) protrusive contact positions and excursions, and (6) the rest position.

Remember that 'positions' refer to mandibular–maxillary relationships, while 'occlusion' refers to tooth-to-tooth relationships.

Intercuspal position (ICP)

The ICP will be approximately 1 mm anterior to the RCP in 90% of the population. Decide whether or not the occlusion and position are acceptable. Acceptability is determined according to:

Function
The occlusion may be functionally unacceptable usually as a result of tooth

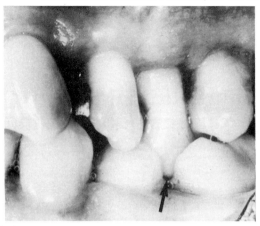

Fig. 4.1 This occlusion requires modification in the intercuspal position because the over-erupted |5 is acting as a 'plunger' between |46—and the patient complained of food packing. (Courtesy of Mr V. J. Ward.)

loss and over-eruption (fig. 4.1). Alteration by means of tooth reshaping or restoration may be necessary. However a malaligned intercuspal position occlusion may be functionally acceptable (see fig 1.6).

Aesthetics

Figure 4.2 shows a patient whose acquired intercuspal position is aesthetically and functionally unacceptable to him.

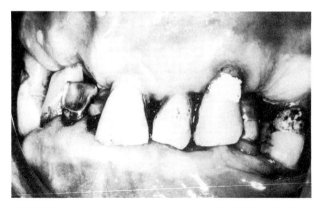

Fig. 4.2 The intercuspal position required modification for both aesthetic and functional reasons.

Traumatic relationships

Between: (1) Tooth and opposing soft tissue which may sometimes be alleviated by adjustment of the intercuspal position (however, see fig. 4.3); (2) Teeth, resulting in either wear, mobility, drifting or mechanical failures (figs 4.4(*a*) and (*b*)). The alteration of the intercuspal position (by occlusal adjustment, restoration or orthodontics) would result in a more acceptable tooth relationship.

Adaptation to wear

Although eruption may occur together with attrition, the resulting relationships in the ICP may not enable the dentist to provide restorations because of inadequate crown height (see fig. 3.15). Sometimes the ICP requires modification, either by adjustment to the retruded position or by small alterations of vertical dimension to allow for placement of restorative materials. The latter procedure must be done with caution and only following a trial period of temporary restorations.

Intercuspal position acceptable

If restorations are required and the dentist decides that the intercuspal position is acceptable, he must ensure that the restorations reproduce the existing position accurately, because alterations should be prescribed and planned and not haphazard. The techniques available will be described in Chapter 7.

Retruded contact position (RCP)

The significance of contacts on the retruded arc of movement are closely related to the findings described in Chapter 3.

Mobility

In the absence of pocketing, but in the presence of muscle sensitivity, a tooth which is mobile and is the initial contact in the RCP will probably tighten after occlusal adjustment.

Bruxism

Several authors[1-3] believe that adjustment of contacts in the RCP to achieve even contact between multiple teeth in this relationship and eliminating the 'slide' from RCP to ICP will eliminate bruxism. Further work is required to substantiate this claim.

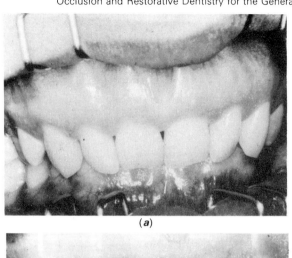

(a)

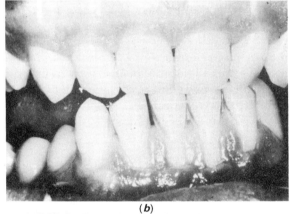

(b)

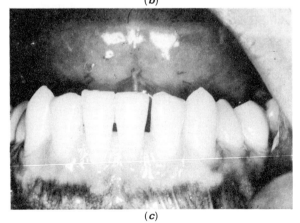

(c)

Fig. 4.3 The patient who had a Class II, division 2 occlusion, was referred to his dentist because of 'stripping of the gingivae' (**a**) and (**b**). However, note (**c**) the tissue after *only* scaling, polishing and plaque control. No occlusal adjustment was necessary. Therefore if traumatic relationship is the provisional diagnosis, always remove plaque induced inflammation and then reassess. (Courtesy Mr J. B. Kieser.)

Adaptation

Deflective contacts in the retruded position may lead to a path of closure which avoids these single tooth contacts, that is, the intercuspal position may depend on avoidance of RCP contacts. Figures 4.5(*a*) and (*b*) show the important difference between the retruded contact position and contact in the intercuspal position.

Consider a tooth which is to be restored and is an initial contact in the retruded position. Elimination of the occlusal surface during tooth preparation may result in an alteration of the intercuspal position, there no longer being any need to avoid the deflective, retruded occlusal contact. However, there is insufficient experimental data to allow the clinician to determine with confidence when such an alteration will occur.

The first possibility to be considered is that the tooth or teeth to be prepared are not initial contacts in the retruded position (figs 4.6(*a*)–(*c*)). Clearance between prepared occlusal surface and opposing teeth can be predicted: that is, if 1 mm of occlusal tissue is removed, 1 mm of clearance results (fig. 4.6(*c*)).

The second possibility is that the tooth or teeth to be prepared are initial contacts in the retruded position (fig. 4.6(*d*)). In this case the possible results are:

ICP retained   The mandible may continue to move to the original ICP on closure (fig. 4.6(*e*)).

Immediate adaptation   During tooth preparation the initial contacts are inadvertently removed (fig. 4.6(*a*)). There is an immediate adaptive res-

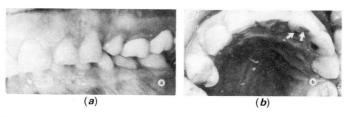

| (*a*) | (*b*) |

Fig. 4.4(*a*) Intercuspal position. |1 exhibits grade II mobility and the patient report that it 'felt heavy since his dentist cemented the crowns', (**b**) Showing fractured porcelain |1 coinciding with ICP contact against |1.

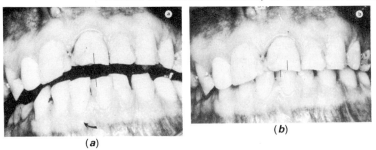

(b)

(a)

Fig. 4.5(a) The RCP. (**b**) The ICP. Note that this position is forwards and to the right relative to the RCP.

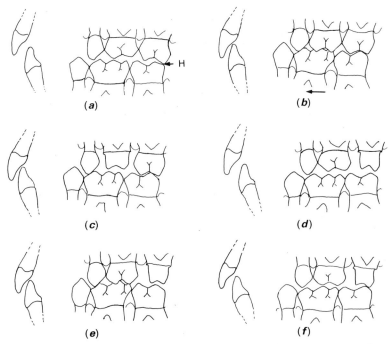

Fig. 4.6(a)–(c) Diagrams to illustrate several possibilities when crown preparations are made. (**a**) RCP—initial contact $\underline{7}\,\overline{7}$ (H). (**b**) ICP—the mandible is more anterior than in **a**, avoiding the deflective contact between $\underline{7}\,\overline{7}$. (**c**), $\underline{6}$ prepared for crown, the deflective contact has not been touched and therefore the ICP is retained. (**d**) $\underline{7}$ prepared for crown: in so doing the deflective contact has been removed. (**e**) The original ICP may be retained, and there is room for the restoration. (**f**) Adaptation may occur: the mandible moving along a new path of closure, resulting in insufficient room for the restoration.

ponse, such that the mandible now closes slightly distally to the original intercuspal position, because the deflective occlusal contact has been removed (fig. 4.6(*f*)). The dentist may instruct the patient to 'close' and find that although he removed, say, 1 mm of tooth structure, only 0·25 mm of occlusal clearance occurs, because of the distal mandibular repositioning. This may also be accompanied by superior positioning of the condyle resulting in even less clearance between opposing teeth (fig. 4.6(*f*)). This is particularly liable to occur when the last tooth in the arch is prepared.

Delayed adaptation during temporary phase of treatment The teeth are prepared and temporary restorations placed. The patient maintains the original intercuspal position. Owing to the poor abrasion resistance of plastic temporary materials and the difficulty of reproducing accurately the original occlusal form, mandibular repositioning may occur. The patient may frequently return with the temporaries uncemented, fractured or high and each time they are replaced the occlusion is again changed (combination of fig. 4.6(*e*) and (*f*)). On trying in the final restorations, these may be found to be high and the dentist blames the technician for incompetence. However, the error was his, since he did not recognise the problem prior to tooth preparation.

If the temporary restorations are made out of occlusion, mandibular repositioning may occur without any occlusal discomfort, however when the final restorations are placed these may again be high.

If the tooth to be prepared is the initial contact in the retruded position, it is prudent to investigate the occlusion further and adjust the occlusal contacts on this tooth prior to preparation. Only proceed with crown preparations when posterior stability can be assured, following removal of occlusal tissue. This is particularly significant if the tooth to be prepared is at the end of the arch or if entire quadrants are to be restored since the resistance to condylar repositioning under the influence of the muscles is eliminated.

If the patient exhibits muscle tenderness and temporary bridge work is required at an early stage of treatment, it is prudent to adjust the occlusion on the temporaries until the muscle tenderness has been eliminated and the mandible exhibits free arcing movements about the retruded axis. Only then can the impressions and jaw registrations be made with confidence. Sometimes the adjustment on the temporaries (better termed provisional restorations) can take 6 to 9 months and in these circumstances it is frequently better to make cast metal or acrylic reinforced by cast metal restorations.

Deflective contacts should never be introduced, but commonly are by restoration, orthodontic therapy, poor occlusal adjustment, dentures, unopposed over-erupted teeth, corrective jaw surgery with inadequate post-operative occlusal adjustments or restoration, or tilting of teeth.

Deflective contacts may be inadvertently removed by occlusal adjustment, orthodontic movement, surgical repositioning, tooth preparation for a restoration, or extraction.

Slide from RCP to ICP

If restorations are required in the presence of a slide, the dentist must decide whether to:

(1) Restore to ICP, ensuring that new deflective contacts are not introduced into the restorations thereby altering the slide.

(2) Eliminate the slide and restore to RCP.

(3) Eliminate the slide and restore to RCP, leaving an area of freedom in the restorations so that the patient can continue to function in the original ICP.

The advantages of restoring to the RCP are six-fold:

(1) It is a relatively reproducible position, which means that following occlusal adjustments removal of occlusal material during tooth preparation will not result in mandibular repositioning with associated decrease in the interocclusal clearance between prepared teeth.

(2) The operator can manipulate the mandible to the desired vertical dimension and establish tooth-to-tooth contacts without patient interference. He is therefore able to establish occlusal contacts in the restorations which obtain the maximum potential from the remaining tooth tissue or restorative materials by controlling the location and direction of occlusal loads.

(3) Evenness of occlusal contacts can be provided because the operator can establish and test contacts without patient guidance.

(4) All movements occur anterior to the RCP, and so the clinician can have control, if he so desires, of potential contacting surfaces.

(5) It is a position the patient can attain, but it is not necessarily physiologically correct for all people. The position may be more of mechanical convenience than physiological correctness.[4]

(6) The retruded contact position can be transferred to an articulator, and small changes in vertical dimension accurately made, if necessary, such that tooth-to-tooth contacts established will be the same as those in the patient's mouth. Thus, it is a useful reference and starting point for restoration.

The findings of the examination will determine the choice of RCP or ICP for fabrication of restorations. Whenever the slide from RCP to ICP is to be eliminated it is imperative that this be carried out prior to definitive tooth preparation, by either occlusal adjustment or placement of temporary restorations (provisionals) and their adjustment. Adjustment is continued until the RCP is clinically reproducible. Only then can the restoration be carried out with confidence. (The term reproducible related to RCP is relative, since many studies have demonstrated that different RCPs can be established by different techniques.) It is now generally conceded that the condyles in the RCP are superiorly positioned with their anterior surfaces seated by way of the disc against the posterior slope of the eminentia[4] (fig. 4.7).

Significance of the direction of the slide

Anterior slide is when the slide from the RCP to the ICP is straight forward. If the tooth to be prepared is uninvolved in the sliding contacts, ensure that the restoration does not alter the situation. If the tooth to be restored is the deflective contact inducing the slide, it is important to adjust the occlusion on this tooth prior to restoration to ensure that removal of occlusal tissue during preparation will not result in mandibular repositioning (fig. 4.6). This becomes even more significant when an entire quadrant is to be restored. Alternatively the cuspal inclines must be accurately reproduced in both the temporary and final restorations, to reproduce the slide—a difficult exercise.

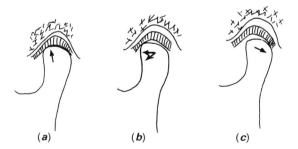

(a)   (b)   (c)

Fig. 4.7 Diagram to represent condylar positions. (*a*) In the RCP the condyle is positioned superiorly with its anterior surface seated by way of the disc (*shaded*) against the posterior facing slope of the eminence. (*b*) The condyle is not superiorly positioned. (*c*) The condyle is retruded (by the dentist) but not superiorly positioned (*b*) and (*c*) are incorrect.

Lateral slide (fig. 4.5)   If the slide from RCP to ICP is forwards and to one side, or just to one side, then this should usually be eliminated prior to restoration. However, this can be qualified further by stating that elimination should be considered if:

(1) The tooth to be restored is a deflective contact.
(2) The tooth to be restored is at the end of the slide, that is $\lfloor\underline{1}$ is to have PJC and $\lfloor\underline{1}$ exhibits fremitus caused by the slide from RCP to ICP.
(3) An entire quadrant is to be restored.
(4) The entire dentition is to be restored.

Significance of the nature of the slide

The motion is divided into vertical and horizontal components. A slide with a large vertical but small horizontal dimension is easy to adjust whereas one with a large horizontal but small vertical dimension is difficult to adjust.

Large vertical but small horizontal dimension   It can be seen from figure 4.8 that if the mandible were to move downwards along the retruded arc of movement, the effect of arcing would move the lower incisors distally in relation to the maxillary incisors as the vertical dimension increased. Therefore, if cuspal contacts were such that the RCP were associated with a large increase in vertical dimension as compared to the ICP, the distal relationship of the lower anterior teeth to the upper anteriors could be due largely to the arcing effect. The actual bodily distal shift of the mandible relative to the maxilla would be minimal. Figure 4.9 shows the ICP and RCP positions in which the apparent distal positioning of the lower anterior teeth is due mainly to altered vertical dimension in the RCP and

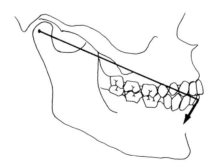

Fig. 4.8 As opening occurs about the retruded axis, the effect of arcing moves the lower incisors distally relative to the uppers (*arrow*).

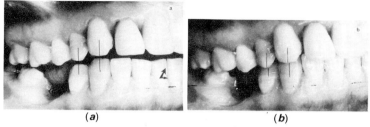

(a)   (b)

Fig. 4.9(a) The RCP. (b) The ICP in a patient with a large vertical, but small horizontal dimension between the two positions. The lines on the canines and first premolars indicate the amount of anterior movement from RCP to the ICP.

the effect of arcing. Adjustment of the deflective contact in such a case would result in the adjusted RCP being almost coincident with the ICP.

This type of involvement is relatively easy since there are few cusps involved which being large can be seen readily. The patient will tend to adapt to the adjusted position rapidly, since it will be almost coincident with the ICP. Slight overclosure with the adjustment will make the adjusted RCP and ICP even closer provided there is no lateral component to the slide.

Large horizontal but small vertical dimension between RCP and ICP. If the mandible were distally displaced by 1 mm from the ICP (fig. 4.10) with little or no increase in vertical dimension, the discrepancy between the upper and lower anterior teeth when RCP is compared to ICP would be actual, owing to a true distal positioning of the mandible. Figure 4.11 shows the RCP and ICP where such a situation is present. Occlusal adjustment in this case may be difficult since many cusps would be involved with only small slides present on each incline. Following adjustment, the new RCP will be distal to the ICP and the operator would not know

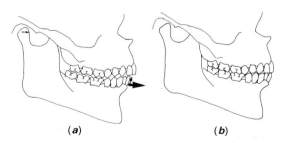

(a)   (b)

Fig. 4.10 Diagrammatic representation of large horizontal but small vertical dimension between (a) RCP and (b) ICP.

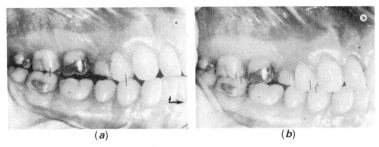

(a)   (b)

Fig. 4.11(a) The RCP (b) The ICP in a patient with a large horizontal but small vertical dimension between the RCP and ICP. The lines on the first premolars and second molars indicate the horizontal discrepancy.

whether the patient would function in the adjusted position, the previous intercuspal position or somewhere in between. If a new position were adopted, then large horizontal rubbing surfaces would have been created on the posterior teeth which can be difficult to accommodate, can give rise to squeaking sounds, and can make anterior guidance difficult to provide since it may result in elimination of contact between upper and lower anterior teeth. The general practitioner should concentrate his efforts on the large vertical with small horizontal slide until he is proficient in the management of such cases before progressing to the large horizontal with small vertical type.

Dimensions of the slide from RCP to ICP
Small slides may be easy to adjust, but large slides, common in the Class II division 1 case, may be difficult to adjust and obtain patient comfort, and in these situations it may be better to restore the existing ICP, taking great care to ensure that it is copied accurately.

Ease of slide
If the patient has freedom between the RCP and the ICP, but there is no inclined plane action forcing the mandible into the ICP, then restorations should copy the existing relationships.

Lateral positions and excursions

Working side contacts
Tooth contacts in lateral excursion are particularly important during bruxist activity, since restorations may alter the direction of mandibular movement in such activity, leading to mechanical failures or discomfort.

Mandibular movement is guided by condyle–fossa relationships and tooth relationships. When the tooth guidance is from the front of the mouth, this is termed anterior guidance, that is, the influence on mandibular movement of contacting surfaces of anterior teeth. Some authors believe that the guidance in the lateral excursion should be only on the canines, whereas others believe that there should be multiple contact on the working side, known as 'group function'. A combination suggested by others is one in which guidance commences as group function and continues as canine guidance. The three concepts have in common the proviso that non-working side interferences are eliminated. In the absence of signs or symptoms, it is best to copy the existing guidance when restorations are required. Whenever the guiding surfaces are to be incorporated into restorations the following principles should be used:

(1) Lateral movements should be smooth.

(2) Use similar materials between opposing contacting surfaces, if possible, to control wear with the subsequent changing guidance (fig. 4.12), or failure of restorative material through exposure of cement.

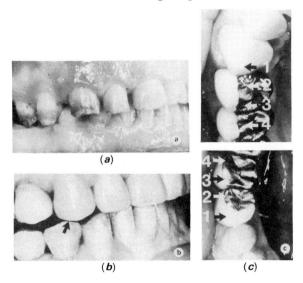

(a)

(b)   (c)

Fig. 4.12 Control of excursive contacts. (*a*) Before treatment, advanced wear. (*b*) Guidance has been arranged as follows. 3|3 were uncrowned. In right latero-protrusive movements (midway between straight protrusion and right lateral) porcelain on the mesial of 4| (contact 1 (*c*)) contacts porcelain on the distal of 3|. Dentine of 321| contacted porcelain on 21|1. If the dentine wears, guidance should be maintained on the porcelain 3| 4|. In protrusion and right lateral excursion there is a similar arrangement. However, 54| 54| are arranged such that (*c*) if the porcelain to porcelain 3| 4| contact 1 wears or 3| moves, 54| 54| will drop into group function with gold contacts 2,3,4 against gold.

(3) Eliminate non-working side contacts (discussed below).

(4) Ensure that there is no excessive movement of the guiding teeth, unless this is due to the reduced but healthy periodontium. In these circumstances, splinting may sometimes be required to stabilise the guiding teeth.

(5) If existing mandibular movement does not fulfil the above requirements, adjustment may be necessary prior to restoration.

(6) If change is necessary or guidance unknown, it is usually 'mechanically' easier to create the guidance as far forwards as possible—on the canines and premolars rather than the molars.

Non-working side contacts

According to most workers, non-working side contacts are particularly significant because of their destructive nature. The potential for damaging the masticatory apparatus has been attributed[5] to: changes in the mandibular leverage; the placement of forces outside the long axes of the teeth; and disruption of normal muscle function.

It can be seen from figure 3.6 (Part 3) that the presence of non-working side contacts can transfer the guidance on the non-working side from the condyle against the fossa to cusp against the cusp. If the teeth to be restored are non-working side contacts, elimination of occlusal tissue for preparation will alter the guidance of the mandible, and it may not be possible to eliminate these contacts on the subsequent restorations. Non-working side contacts are particularly significant if associated with lateral pterygoid sensitivity on the same side, in which case adjustment of these contacts prior to restoration is essential. Non-working side interferences can affect the anterior teeth as shown in figure 4.13.

Most dentists, in fact, eliminate non-working side contacts on their amalgam restorations, since they automatically instruct their patients to move their jaws from side to side after placement of the restoration, and any lateral contacts are ground out of the amalgam by the dentist. They do this knowing that the presence of these contacts will result in fracture of the restorations. This will be further considered in Chapter 6.

Protrusive positions and excursions

All modern theories of occlusion state that in protrusion the tooth contact should be in the anterior portion of the mouth, with separation of posterior teeth. An occlusion requiring restoration, particularly of the anterior teeth, should be investigated for protrusive contacts because posterior protrusive interferences must be eliminated prior to restoration of the anterior teeth (fig. 4.14).

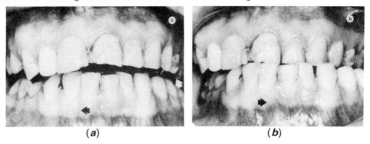

(a)   (b)

Fig. 4.13 Effect of posterior contacts on anterior teeth. (*a*) Right latero-protrusion: a non-working side contact between |7 |7 (*white arrow*) separates the 321| 321|, allowing 321| to over-erupt. (*b*) Left latero-protrusion: Anterior contact prevents over-eruption and allows wear to occur on the upper incisal edges. The net result is uneven incisal edges.

As in the case of a non-working side interference, a posterior protrusive interference can result in over-eruption of an anterior tooth. When anterior teeth are to be crowned, the dentist must decide whether he is to copy the existing anterior guidance, or alter it.

The existing guidance should be copied if there is either an absence of signs or symptoms (the anterior teeth merely requiring crowns) or, in the presence of an adaptive occlusion in the ageing patient, for whom only anterior crowns are required.

Alteration of the anterior guidance may be necessary in the presence of either signs and symptoms of occlusal disturbance manifested in the anterior teeth, or sometimes in full mouth rehabilitation.

If the guidance is to be changed, the dentist must prescribe the shape of

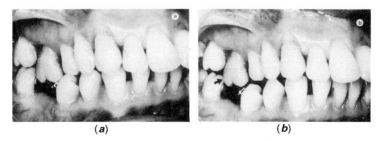

(a)   (b)

Fig. 4.14 Posterior protrusive interference. (*a*) The ICP. (*b*) Protrusion: in protrusion the over-erupted 6| contacts the 7| separating the anterior teeth. The posterior contact must be adjusted prior to any necessary crown restoration of the upper anterior teeth, otherwise the technician may match the anterior guidance to this posterior guidance. Consider the aesthetic implications—the anteriors would be made too long. Also consider the occlusal effect if the adjustment was not carried out and the 6| was subsequently extracted or shortened.

the lingual concavity of the anterior teeth, that is, prescribe the anterior guidance. This will be further discussed in Chapter 9, on anterior restorations. The same criteria described for lateral excursions can be applied to protrusive and latero-protrusive movements: the movement should be smooth; similar materials used if possible; absence of protrusive interferences; and no excessive movement of guidance teeth.

The rest position

Average figures for interocclusal clearance are meaningless. As a general rule try and work within 0·5 mm of the existing vertical dimension in the intercuspal position. If change is necessary for aesthetics or to provide space for restorative materials or for function, then always eliminate deflective contacts between RCP and ICP, and test the change in vertical dimension on diagnostic appliances, such as removable splints, amalgams or temporary crowns (fig. 4.15).

Remember, in wear cases, some of the lost vertical dimension may have been replaced by compensatory mechanisms.

Special investigations

Mounted casts
Casts mounted on a semi-adjustable articulator enable the dentist to observe the occlusal contacts readily (fig. 4.16). The procedures will be described in Chapter 5.

Diagnostic waxing
This will frequently provide invaluable information with regard to aesthetics, tooth contour, the feasibility of occlusal adjustment, nature of tooth preparations, the need for resective periodontal procedures (crown-lengthening procedures), and orthodontic treatment.

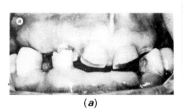 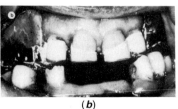

(a)   (b)

Fig. 4.15(a) Advanced wear. (b) Removable appliance to test increased vertical dimensions. Deflective RCP contacts were removed. Cold cure acrylic was added until the patient was at his most comfortable and aesthetic vertical dimension.

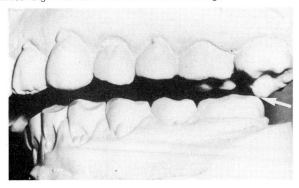

Fig. 4.16 Diagnostic casts in the RCP. Initial contact is between the unopposed over-erupted $\overline{7}$ $\overline{6}$. Always check unopposed molars, particularly 8|8. (These casts correspond to figure 1.1 (*d*)–(*f*). Note that the upper anterior crowns had been provided without removing the deflective posterior contact.)

Pantographic survey

The inability to obtain reproducible pantographic tracings from one day to the next is an indication of muscle dysfunction, and complex restorations should not be carried out in these circumstances.

Conclusion

The clinical significance of the occlusal aspect of the examination has been described, and further consideration of restorative techniques will be discussed in Chapters 6 to 9. The occlusal findings become more significant in the presence of muscle sensitivity. With practice, the discerning dentist will be able to decide which patients require simple management of their occlusions and for which patients a more complex approach is necessary.

References

1 Ramfjord S P. Dysfunctional temporomandibular joint and muscle pain. *J Prosthet Dent* 1961; **11**: 353–374.
2 Dawson P E. *Evaluation, diagnosis and treatment of occlusal problems*, p. 103. St Louis: C V Mosby, 1974.
3 Solberg W K, Woo M W, Houston J B. Prevalence of signs and symptoms of mandibular dysfunction. *J Dent Res* 1975; **54a**: Abst. 432, 153.
4 Celenza F V. Position paper In *Occlusion, the state of the art*, Celenza F V, Nasedkin J N (ed), p 35. Chicago. Quintessence, 1978.
5 Shillingburg H T, Hobo S, Whitsett L D. *Fundamentals of fixed prosthodontics*, p 53. Chicago: Quintessence, 1978.

5 Principles and Types of Articulator with Techniques for Recording Jaw Positions

The main types of articulator are considered together with their clinical use. The type of jaw registration used to mount casts in an articulator partly depends upon whether the mounting is for diagnosis or restoration—both types are described.

A dental articulator is defined in the glossary of prosthodontic terms[1] as a 'mechanical device which represents the temporomandibular joint and jaw members, to which maxillary and mandibular casts may be attached'.

If dental casts are accurately attached to an articulator, it is possible to simulate certain occlusal relationships. The facility of articulators to reproduce these relationships accurately depends on their adjustability and this will be discussed later.

Application of dental articulators

Articulators are used for:

(1) *Diagnosis* enables the dentist to observe various occlusal relationships. It also enables him to carry out diagnostic waxing and tooth repositioning on casts with some degree of accuracy.

(2) *Restoration* Articulators facilitate the development of both the occlusion and aesthetics.

The occlusion
The articulator allows the dentist and technician to produce the prescribed occlusal surfaces accurately. The extent to which the instrument is used, depends upon the number and complexity of restorations and the exper-

ience of both dentist and technician. A single restoration constructed on hand-held casts may take 5 minutes to 'grind-in in the mouth'. Four restorations similarly constructed may require an hour and exhibit none of the occlusal requirements for restorations, as described below. With 16 restorations it may not be possible to adjust in the mouth satisfactorily.

Until the dentist is able to produce smooth tooth preparations, good impressions, good tissue management and accurate jaw registrations, and the technician is able to produce well-contoured, accurately fitting castings on well-prepared dies and casts, the use of sophisticated articulators and the treatment of complex cases, should not be undertaken. The dentist and technician should work jointly using simple devices and gradually progress to more complex procedures as they develop an understanding of the various instruments.

Aesthetics

By relating working casts precisely to the horizontal plane (assuming the patient is sitting upright; fig. 5.1) the technician is able to achieve a better sense of perspective, which will prevent the production of restorations with incorrect occlusal planes (fig. 5.2).

Before describing the types of articulators available and their uses, an understanding of jaw registration is necessary.

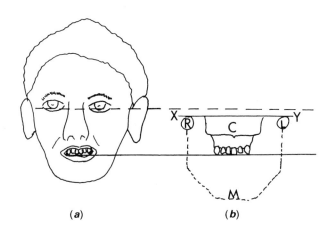

(a)   (b)

Fig. 5.1(a) Patient. (b) Articulator. The upper cast can be mounted with reference to the horizontal plane. XY=Axis of articulator. LR=Left and right articulator condyles. C=Upper cast. M=Mandibular portion of the articulator.

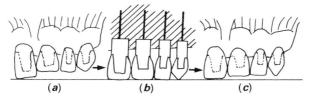

Fig. 5.2 Diagrammatic representation of possible aesthetic errors if the cast is not mounted with reference to the horizontal plane. (*a*) Original tooth outline plus outlined preparations; note |123 are short. (*b*) Dies on working cast. The technician is requested to make the incisal edges straight. Since he has no information about the horizontal, he assumes that the incisal edges of the preparations should be horizontal. (*c*) Note the effect when the crowns are returned to the mouth. The dentist unfairly blames the technician.

REGISTRATION FOR DIAGNOSIS

The main reason for mounting study casts for diagnostic purposes are: to investigate further the initial contacts in the retruded contact position, the slide from the retruded to the intercuspal position, and lateral-occlusal contacts. To achieve the first two it is essential to make a jaw registration on the retruded arc of movement prior to tooth contact, that is a tooth-apart jaw registration. This eliminates the proprioceptive effect of tooth contacts. Lateral contacts require lateral registrations.

Techniques for obtaining retruded diagnostic jaw registrations

Many techniques have been advocated and described and the technique chosen depends partly on the dentist's experience, and partly on the degree of difficulty in occlusal registration. Some patients will exhibit retruded jaw movements with ease, whereas others require a period of deconditioning prior to registration. As stated previously it is essential that the posterior teeth do not contact during the jaw registration technique. Regardless of the method, records should be as thin as possible.

Registration technique for patients who 'exhibit easy movement on the retruded arc of movement'

Equipment
  Wax: Moyco Beauty Pink hard wax, which softens at 55°C
  Soft metal No. 10
  Scissors

Water bath, for maintaining the wax temperature at 55°C (if unavailable use warm water in a bowl, but this is not so dependable)
Bowl of cold water preferably iced
Scalpel with No. 11 blade

Technique The wax is warmed in the water bath to 55°C and a section of soft metal cut so as to be twice the length from first premolar to second molar and narrower than the dimension of lower premolar to premolar across the arch. The wax is removed from the bath, the metal folded over the back of the wax and the wax folded back over the metal (fig. 5.3(a)). The wax is then taken to the mouth or study cast and pressed against the maxillary teeth (fig. 5.3(b)). It is then removed and trimmed with the scissors so that it extends only to the tips of the upper buccal cusps (fig. 5.3(c)). The wax is replaced in the water bath and re-heated. The patient is placed in the recumbent position, and the dentist checks for ease of mandibular manipulation of the mandible to the retruded position, as described in Chapter 2.

The bilateral manipulation technique is the method of choice. After rehearsal the patient is instructed in the following procedure: the wax is removed from the water bath and placed against the upper teeth; the mandible is manipulated to the retruded position and 'jiggled briefly' to ensure ease of movement, and then held in the retruded position while the chairside assistant gently blows air over the wax to chill. On removal from the mouth, the wax is checked for perforations which would indicate tooth-to-tooth contact (fig. 5.3(d)). If satisfactory, it is placed into the iced water. After chilling for a while it is positioned on the maxillary teeth again, to ensure that no distortion has occurred and then on the study casts (if available) to check for accuracy of seating (fig. 5.3(e)).

Techniques for patients with 'moderate difficulty in manipulation of the mandible'

Anterior stop techniques
It is easier to record the retruded axis position if some form of platform is placed against the anterior teeth with the mandible in the retruded position, the lower incisors may close up against this platform and thus prevent posterior tooth contacts (fig. 5.4). This allows the dentist to insert the recording medium between the posterior teeth and readily hold the mandible against the anterior stop while the recording medium sets. The four functions of the stop, are to:
● 'Break proprioceptive reflexes'.

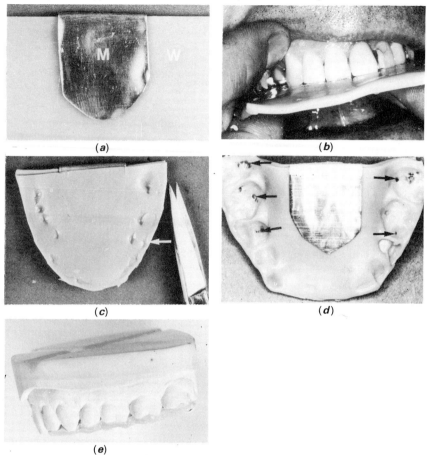

Fig. 5.3 Stages in making a retruded jaw registration without tooth contact. (*a*) Metal (M) folded over warmed wax (W). (*b*) Warm wax pressed against maxillary teeth. (*c*) Trimming wax to extend to the tips of the buccal cusps (further trimming is required). (*d*) Perforated wax (*arrows*) indicates tooth contact—this cannot be used for diagnostic mounting. (*e*) Checking the chilled wax registration on the cast.

● Facilitate location of the retruded position.
● Enable the mandible to be stabilised during registration.
● Maintain the mandibular–maxillary position with posterior teeth just out of contact thus enabling the posterior record to be as thin as possible.

With this technique, the choice of jaw registration materials becomes more varied, since the anterior stop maintains the vertical dimension during jaw registration. However, a material which is mucostatic during

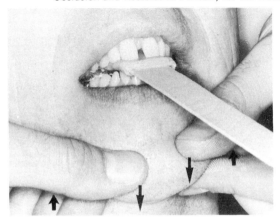

Fig. 5.4 Tongue spatula and wax interior jig plus jaw registration.

insertion and which sets to be rigid and dimensionally stable is the material of choice for the following reasons: since it is mucostatic, it will not displace mobile teeth; being mucostatic, it will not act as an interference resulting in a new proprioceptive reflex; by being rigid it cannot be easily distorted during mounting of casts; by being stable it will not distort during storage. (Wax is a poor material to use if any delay is anticipated between making a registration and mounting the casts.)

The two anterior stops found to be most suitable are a tongue spatula with wax and an acrylic resin jig.

Tongue spatula with wax
This technique is applicable to patients who exhibit slight difficulty in producing the retruded arc of closure (fig. 5.4). Equipment is as before plus: tongue spatula, bite registration paste, or preferably zinc oxide and eugenol temporary cement, such as Temp Bond,[11] spatula for mixing paste or cement.

Technique A piece of hard wax 10 cm by 30 cm is softened at 55°C and wrapped around one end of a wooden tongue spatula. The spatula is placed against the palatal surface of the upper incisors, and the wax moulded over the edges to aid retention. The mandible is then manipulated to the retruded position until the incisal edges of the lower teeth just contact the wax, which is then cooled with air. The indentations of the lower incisors are then trimmed away.

The spatula is replaced and the position is maintained for approximately 5 minutes, which is a reasonable time for the patient to forget, as it were, the habitual position of the mandible and thus facilitate manipulation. The mandible may need to be manipulated several times to ascertain that the lower incisors contact the same areas on the wax stop and ensure reproducibility of the retruded axis position. When the operator is satisfied that this can be achieved, the occlusal registration in wax may be obtained as described previously. The wax wafer must be trimmed anteriorly to accommodate the anterior stop which is retained throughout the entire procedure. When the operator is satisfied that a correct record has been obtained, the wax is removed when hard and finally chilled in iced water. It is then blown dry and a small amount of bite registration paste or Temp Bond is mixed and placed in the impressions made by the cusps of the upper and lower canines, or first premolar and first molars (fig. 5.5). Ensure that space is available for the paste by trimming the wax or by instructing the patient to close into the softened wax with tongue spatula removed before chilling as above. Some paste is also spread over the palatal portion. It is only necessary to capture the tips of the cusps in registration paste to ensure an accurate mounting of casts. The wax registration is replaced in the mouth and the mandible manipulated again and held against the anterior stop until the paste sets. The record is removed and the casts mounted.

If any distortion of the wax registration occurs during mounting of the casts the brittle set paste on the palatal portion will crack, serving as a reliable distortion indicator.

Anterior acrylic jig
This technique is applicable in cases where recording of the retruded position is anticipated to be more difficult than can be managed with the tongue spatula method.

Technique   The making of the jig has been described in Chapter 2, and it is positioned on the upper anterior teeth in the same manner as the tongue spatula. However, it is usually left in place as long as half an hour before jaw registration. (Let the patient sit in the waiting room.)

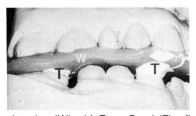

Fig. 5.5 Wax registration (W) with Temp Bond (T) refinement on casts.

Technique for patients with 'greater difficulty in manipulation of the mandible'

The occlusal splint technique is especially useful for those with muscular dysfunction. Many types of occlusal splint have been described and discussed in the literature and reviewed by Zarb and Speck.[2] However, the type that the author prefers is an upper appliance having full occlusal coverage (fig. 5.6). It is designed so as to obtain:

● Even simultaneous contact of all lower posterior teeth against the appliance, in the retruded position. (Note that this position will change as appliance therapy proceeds.)

● Clearance of about 15 μm between the tips of the lower anterior teeth and the appliance (tested with a shimstock) in the retruded position.

● Smooth anterior guidance in excursive movements.

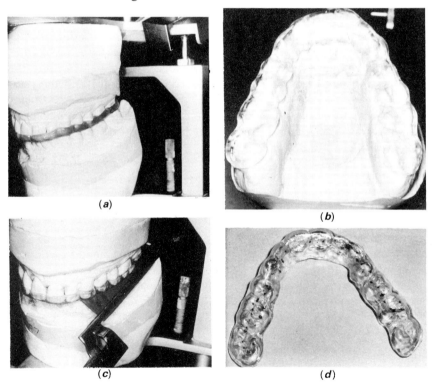

(a)

(b)

(c)

(d)

Fig. 5.6 Occlusal splint. (a) Wax pattern made on mounted casts. (b) Processed splint, not removed from cast. (c) Checking the occlusal contacts. (d) Adjusted splint: ICP/RCP contacts, but absence of posterior working and non-working side contacts.

● Posterior disclusion in excursive movements (absence of posterior contacts during excursive movements).

Technique   The appliance is made from cold cure acrylic on a duplicate upper cast, mounted in an articulator with as good a retruded record as is simply produced. It is first waxed and then the wax converted to plastic. Block out undercuts and have the appliance lip over the incisal edge of the anterior teeth and the buccal and palatal occlusal third of the posteriors. The appliance is inserted and checked for comfort, retention and evenness of occlusal contacts, using occlusal indicating tape in the retruded contact position. Adjustments are made if necessary. The excursions are checked as follows:
● Insert red occlusal tape and instruct the patient to move the mandible in a lateral excursion.
● Remove the red tape and place black tape on posterior occlusal surfaces; guide the patient to tap once in the retruded contact position.
● Remove the appliance and grind away any red posterior marks and irregular anterior marks—adjust the black ones.
● Continue until smooth excursions are obtained in all directions with no posterior contacts during excursions, but with multiple black posterior contacts in the retruded contact position.
It is sometimes necessary to add cold cure acrylic to build up areas of contact.

The appliance is worn, preferably all day and night, until free mandibular movement to the retruded contact position is obtained. It is only removed for cleaning after meals. The above adjustment procedures are repeated frequently because with muscle relaxation the jaw positions will change. Some patients may find it necessary to remove the appliance for meals. It should be checked after 24 hours and again at weekly intervals.

When the operator is satisfied with the ease of mandibular movement, the appliance may be removed taking care not to allow any tooth contact, and an anterior jig inserted before proceeding to register the mandibular--maxillary relationship.

Jaw registration in cases with a posterior edentulous ridge

Prefabricated base plate
Ideally, mounting of casts should be with jaw registration plates, made before the recording session. Study casts are made and these are used as follows:

Technique   Tooth and soft tissue undercuts are blocked out and covered with cold mould seal. Cold cure acrylic is adapted to the cast and built up on the edentulous areas with a brush-on technique. The occlusal surfaces of the teeth are left uncovered. The resultant base-plate should be pressure-polymerised in a Hydroflask. When fully cured it is trimmed and smoothed (fig. 5.7), then checked for fit and retention in the mouth. With the aid of an anterior jig the jaw registration is made as previously described, using registration material over the natural teeth and the built-up area of the acrylic plate which simulates the missing dentition. This is preferable to using the registration plate alone, as any movement of the plate may be detected by its failure to seat in the registration and the cast at the same time.

Posterior teeth missing but registration plate not available
Provided there are sufficient teeth present in the arch to achieve some degree of stability of the wax registration, the tongue spatula with wax technique may be used. However, Temp Bond or bite registration paste should be added to the saddle areas as well as to the teeth (fig. 5.8). Since bite registration paste is mucostatic no distortion of the edentulous ridges will occur and a sufficiently reliable jaw registration for diagnosis may be produced.

Techniques for obtaining lateral and protrusive jaw registrations

Investigation of lateral and protrusive tooth contacts, is also frequently required for diagnosis, and articulators can be programmed by either wax

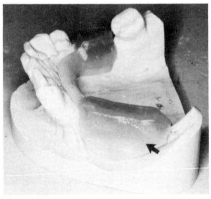

Fig. 5.7 Prefabricated registration plate with wax rims, used for posterior edentulous ridge.

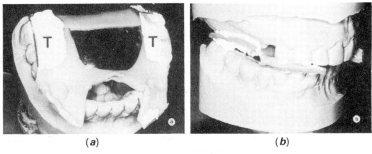

(a)   (b)

Fig. 5.8 Wax and metal jaw registration refined with Temp Bond (T) extended onto the edentulous ridges. (Used when an acrylic registration plate is not available.) (*a*) Palatal surface. (*b*) Mounting the casts.

records, matching facets on the cast, quick analysers, pantographic records, or stereographic records. These techniques will be described subsequently.

REGISTRATION FOR RESTORATION

The most convenient registration for restorative dentistry is that of the intercuspal position, whether this be the existing intercuspal position or the intercuspal position following occlusal adjustment. Wherever possible, the dentist's technique should be developed to utilise an intercuspal relationship. Such registrations are taken with the teeth together at the correct vertical dimension (fig. 5.9). These registrations will be described in Chapter 7.

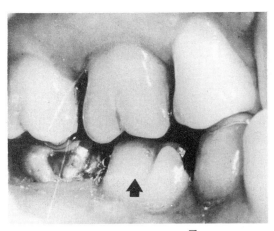

Fig 5.9 Teeth in the ICP showing crown preparation on 6̄|. There are teeth mesial and distal to the preparation, that is it is bounded.

Requirements for dental articulators

It is now possible to consider the requirements of articulators when they are used for diagnosis and for restorations.

Diagnosis

Vertical dimension adjustability to reproduce the RCP   Since diagnostic jaw registrations must be taken at an increased vertical dimension (to prevent posterior tooth contact) it is essential that the articulator be able to close accurately through the thickness of the registration material until tooth contact has occurred. In the retruded position it can be seen (fig. 5.10) that if the axis of rotation of the articulator and the patient do not have the same spatial relationships to the teeth, then closure through the thickness of the registration in the patient would result in a different tooth contact to that which may be seen on the articulator.

Reproduction of lateral and protrusive jaw movements   For the majority of cases great accuracy is not required. However, the instrument should be able to simulate major non-working and posterior protrusive interferences.

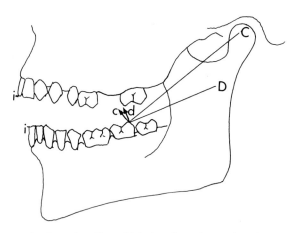

Fig. 5.10 Diagram to show the effect of 'closing through a registration'. i—i=thickness of registration in the incisal region. When the articulator axis corresponds to the patient's axis (C)—note the position of the distal cusp of the over-erupted $\overline{7}$ following removal of the record and closure along the path (c) $\underline{|8}$ is cleared. When the axes do not coincide (D) note the position of $\overline{|7}$ distal cusp following removal of the record and closure along path (d) $\underline{|8}$ is contacted.

Restorations

Vertical dimension adjustability   The need for accuracy following changes in vertical dimension largely depends on the techniques employed by the operator. However, if intercuspal records are used at the correct vertical dimension, there is usually no need to reproduce accurately changes in vertical dimension.

Stability of the mounted position   The articulator must be able to hold the casts accurately in the mounted position when the jaw registration material is removed. Furthermore, following movement of the articulator the casts must be able to return precisely to the original position.

Intercuspal position   If this differs from the mounted position, the articulator should allow the casts to be related in the intercuspal position.

Lateral excursion   The technique employed and the number of teeth to be restored will determine how accurately lateral excursions must be reproduced. This will be discussed shortly.

Aesthetic perspective   When anterior restorations are to be fabricated, it would benefit the technician if the articulator is also capable of providing a perception of anterior aesthetics on the mounted casts.

Types of articulator

Several types of articulator commonly used in the UK will now be considered, relevant to the foregoing considerations. Many of the devices commonly termed articulators are in fact nothing more than cast holders, which do not simulate mandibular movement.

Hand-held casts

The advantages and disadvantages of the hand-held casts shown in figure 5.11 are:
(1) They cannot reproduce the retruded contact position since they cannot be closed accurately through the thickness of a registration once this is removed.
(2) They can reproduce the intercuspal position if sufficient teeth are present.
(3) All lateral and protrusive excursions are guided by the teeth and bear

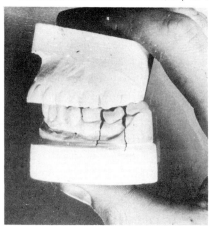

Fig. 5.11 Hand-held casts in the ICP.

no relationship to the joints: they cannot reproduce border movements (defined as any extreme compass of mandibular movement limited by bone, ligaments or soft tissue[1]).

(4) It is difficult to obtain precise contacts during fabrication of restorations, particularly in porcelain, as the restoration is liable to be knocked off if it is high. Inevitably, restorations made on hand-held casts will be out of occlusion.

(5) They are not sufficiently accurate for multiple restorations.

(6) It is not possible to orientate the casts accurately relative to the horizontal plane; therefore the aesthetic perspective is not feasible (consider figure 5.2).

Simple hinge articulators

The simple hinge articulator shown in figure 5.12 is a cast holder, not a proper articulator. Its advantages and disadvantages are:

(1) It cannot be closed accurately through the thickness of a jaw registration, since the relationship of its axis of rotation to the teeth differs to that of the patient; therefore, it is useless for diagnosis of RCP deflective contacts.

(2) There is no facility for accurately altering vertical dimension.

(3) It will hold the intercuspal position if the casts are mounted at the correct vertical dimension and is therefore useful for waxing in the intercuspal position (especially if used with the functionally generated path technique to be described in Chapter 7).

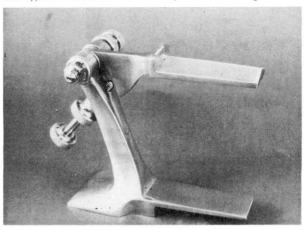

Fig. 5.12 Simple hinge articulator and head.

(4) Lateral and protrusive excursions are inaccurate because the position of the 'condyles' bears no relation to the patient's condyles.

(5) It does not impart aesthetic perspective, as it is used without a facebow.

In clinical use it is valueless for diagnosis. It may be used occasionally for single crowns when the lateral excursions are to be adjusted in the mouth, and may be complimented by the functionally generated path technique. It is useful in the fabrication of temporary crowns. However very little extra time is required to use the semi-adjustable articulator.

Semi-adjustable articulators

There are two types of semi-adjustable articulators: the Arcon (fig. 5.13(*a*)) in which the fossae are on the upper member, and the Non-Arcon (fig. 5.13(*b*)) in which the fossae are on the lower member. Arcon articulators usually have a removable upper member and are good teaching instruments since the joints are the right way round. Theoretically, they are more accurate when setting protrusive angles. However, with non-balanced occlusions this is probably insignificant. If casts are mounted in a Non-Arcon articulator with a retruded record, it may be difficult to position them subsequently in the ICP, since the condyles are locked into the fossa slots.

Facebows

For all types of semi-adjustable articulators closure through the thickness of a jaw registration can be simple and accurate and certainly is acceptable

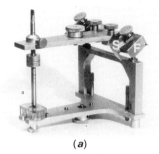 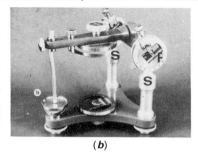

(a)   (b)

5.13 Semi-adjustable articulators. (F=fossa inclination control. S=progressive sideshift control.) (*a*) Arcon articulator (Whipmix). (*b*) Non-Arcon articulator (Dentatus).

for diagnosis. However, this accuracy can only be obtained by using a facebow, of which there are two types, average and kinematic. Either way, the mounted upper cast is related to the articulator joints in a similar way to the relationship between the upper teeth and the patient's joints.

A facebow is a device used to record:

(1) The distance from the joints to the upper teeth (from the retruded axis to the upper teeth is more correct).

(2) The relationship between the axis orbital plane (joining the condylar axis of rotation, with the lower border of the orbit, and corresponds to the Frankfort plane) and the upper occlusal plane (joining the tips of the teeth).

(3) The width between the condyles (on some facebows).

Average facebow

For example the Whipmix facebow which is made up of a bite fork, calipers, earpieces and a nosepiece (fig. 5.14). The bite fork is warmed and covered with wax, and then placed against the upper teeth. It is essential that only the tips of the cusps indent the wax. The remainder of the facebow is assembled according to the manufacturer's instructions and the whole transferred to the articulator (fig. 5.15) to position the upper cast in relation to the articulator's axis of rotation. Thus the cast and condyles of the articulator will be in approximately the same spatial relationship as the upper teeth and condyles of the patient. Following mounting of the upper cast, a retruded jaw registration can be used to orientate the lower cast to it. The lower cast is then fixed to the lower member of the articulator with plaster (fig. 5.16). The lower cast will now be related to the condyles of the articulator as the patient's lower teeth are to his condyles. On removal of the registration the articulator may be closed to observe tooth contacts in the retruded position.

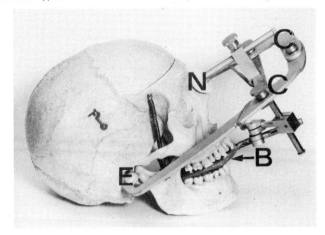

Figure 5.14 Whipmix facebow mounted on a skull. (N=nosepiece-third point of reference. B=bitefork covered with wax and Tempbond reline. E=earpiece. C=calipers.)

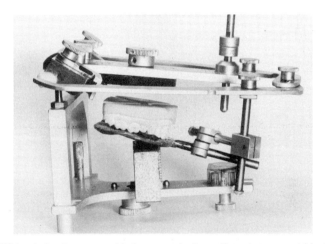

Fig. 5.15 Whipmix facebow assembled on an articulator. Note that support blocks prevent the bitefork from bending under the weight of the cast.

The semi-adjustable articulator used with the average facebow gives a very close approximation, provided the change in vertical dimension on removal of the wax registration is small.

Kinematic facebow

The bow is attached to the lower teeth (fig. 5.17(*a*)) and the mandible

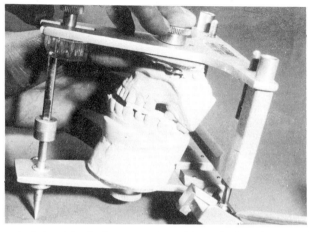

5.16 Lower cast plastered to the lower member of the articulator, by way of a retruded registration. (Articulator inverted for mounting; ensure condyle balls are in fossae.)

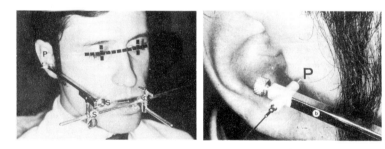

5.17 (*a*) Kinematic facebow used to locate the retruded horizontal axis of rotation (S=vertical and horizontal adjuster). (*b*) Close-up of stylus (P=stylus).

directed along the retruded arc of movement. A point on the horizontal axis of rotation is located with a stylus which is moved by adjustable side-arms. A point is then located on the other side of the face.

A separate bow is used for transferring the spatial relationship to the articulator. The two located points are orientated so as to coincide with the articulator's horizontal axis. Details of the technique have been described by Dawson.[3]

Semi-adjustable articulators when used with a kinematic facebow, give a very accurate reproduction of retruded tooth contacts following the change in vertical dimension resulting from removal of the retruded registration.

Use of semi-adjustable articulators

With either facebow technique, the system is quite acceptable for diagnosis. Arcon semi-adjustable articulators (in particular) are capable of reproducing the intercuspal position following removal of a retruded jaw registration.

For lateral excursions, it is necessary to consider two components of lateral movement: the initial 1 to 2 mm of movement, and movement beyond this.

Initial movement   In most patients lateral movement approximates to a simple rotation about a vertical axis, passing through the condyle on the working side (fig. 5.18(*a*)); whereas for others this condyle may move sideways (fig. 5.18(*b*)) giving rise to immediate side shift. Not only may it move sideways, it may also move upwards and sideways, backwards or forwards and sideways, or any possible combination. Obviously such movement if present will influence tooth contacts. Much discussion has taken place about its cause, significance and nature, whether physiological or pathological. The interested reader is referred to the bibliography in Chapter 10. Some patients may exhibit a combination of rotation and immediate side shift in the initial movement.

Movement beyond the initial 1 to 2 mm (or total movement if no immediate side shift). According to Lundeen and Wirth[4] this movement can be simply described as occurring about a vertical axis in the region of the working side condyle. The movement of the non-working side condyle relative to the sagittal plane can be recorded and the angle set on an articulator so that the instrument reproduces its progressive side shift, that is sideways movement of the mandible occurring at a rate or amount directly proportional to the

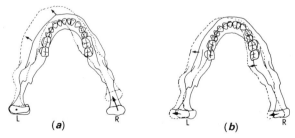

5.18 Diagrammatic representation of left lateral excursion. (*a*) Simple rotation through the left condyle (L=new position, dashed). Note the movement of the right condyle (R). (*b*) Initial sideways movement. New position shown dashed. Note movement of R.

forward movement of the orbiting (non-working) condyle; it is essentially a straight line.[5]

The semi-adjustable articulator approximates lateral excursions, but errors can result from:

(1) A limited ability to adjust progressive side shift.
(2) No facility for reproduction of immediate side shift. (Several of the recent semi-adjustable articulators have average immediate side shift adjustability, for example Denar Mark II and Panadent.)
(3) Limited adjustability for protrusive settings.
(4) Limited or no adjustability of the distance between the condyles.

Use for restorations—for most restorative treatment, the semi-adjustable articulator is the instrument of choice. It is particularly suitable for restorations bounded by teeth on each side (fig. 5.19), and this will be discussed in Chapter 7. Finally, with the use of a facebow the semi-adjustable articulator imparts an aesthetic perspective.

The use of the semi-adjustable articulator for restorative therapy requires a knowledge of occlusion so as to overcome the problems of excursive inaccuracies. This will be further discussed under specific restorations in Chapter 7. It should be used judiciously for wear cases with shallow condylar guidance, and may only be used for full mouth restoration when treatment is divided into four stages:

(1) Stabilisation of jaw relationships, that is elimination of slide from RCP to ICP, followed by

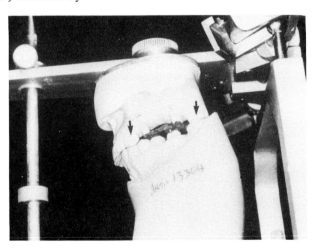

Fig. 5.19 Working casts mounted in Whipmix articulator. The prepared teeth have unprepared teeth both mesially and distally.

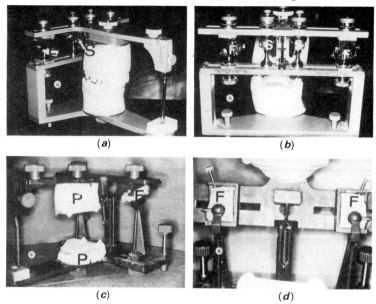

(a)   (b)

(c)   (d)

Fig. 5.20 Examples of two fully adjustable articulators (F=fossa inclination control, S=sideshift control). (*a*) Stuart articulator from side. (*b*) Stuart from behind showing condylar controls. (*c*) TMJ articulator from side (casts are removed although mounting plaster P is present). (*d*) Condylar controls. Fossae are moulded from plastic F.

(2) Determination of the anterior guidance whilst maintaining posterior stability.

(3) Restoration of the anterior segment while maintaining posterior stability.

(4) Restoration of the posterior segments.

Fully-adjustable articulators

These articulators have a large range of adjustability in three dimensions. (Two examples are shown in figure 5.20.)

Their advantages are that they can accurately

(1) Reproduce changes in vertical dimension on the retruded arc of movement.

(2) Reproduce lateral movements in the most posterior range, that is border movements. (They can all reproduce immediate and progressive side shift.)

(3) Return the casts to the mounted relationship (and the intercuspal position, if these differ).

(4) Reproduce the aesthetic perspective (although if, when the patient is upright, the kinematically located axis is not close to the horizontal plane, this could present difficulties).

They are good instruments for diagnosis and restoration, but are not necessary for the majority of restorative work in general practice. Many clinicians would regard the fully-adjustable articulator as essential for full mouth restoration when all the restorations are to be fabricated at the same time, or when complications due to wear, bruxism or shallow condylar or shallow anterior guidance are anticipated. This will be further discussed in Chapters 6 to 9.

The choice of articulator for restorative therapy is partly dependent on the nature of the restorations, the nature of the patient's problem and the experience of the dentist and his technician. Most restorative therapy should be carried out on the semi-adjustable articulator, but the simple hinge articulator may be used with a functionally generated path technique for one to three units. However, when the treatment of complex cases is undertaken the time spent programming the fully adjustable articulators is fully compensated because the bulk of the work is carried out in the laboratory rather than in the patient's mouth. It is far more accurate and less time-consuming to carry out the small occlusal adjustments required following the careful fabrication of restorations on a fully adjustable articulator, than grinding in 32 castings in a patient's mouth following their fabrication on a simple hinge articulator.

Methods of setting lateral and protrusive excursions

Hand-held casts
The only way is to try and match faceting on the opposing teeth. All movement will be tooth-guided.

Simple hinge articulator
Try and match the facets (less accurate than hand-held casts since the 'joint' of the articulator limits the movements). Since the movements are so inaccurate they are of no clinical value.

Semi-adjustable articulator
Wax registrations are made in lateral and protrusive positions (fig. 5.21) and these registrations are then transferred to the casts mounted on the articulator. The condylar elements are then adjusted to enable the records to be seated between the casts. This gives an average path of movement between any two records, but no information about movement between the two.

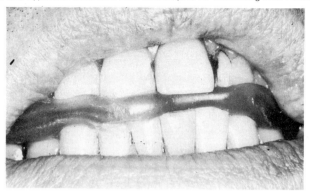

Fig. 5.21 Wax registration being made in protrusive excursion (edge to edge). For lateral registrations the lower incisors are guided approximately 4 mm to the right or left, and the registration made.

Recently, quick analyser systems have been introduced. These are relatively simple tracing devices which indicate the amount of progressive side shift present together with an approximation of immediate side shift. They may become useful diagnostic tools.

Fully adjustable articulators
These articulators can be programmed by two types of records:

Pantographs   A pantographic device (fig. 5.22) is used to record border and protrusive excursions and to transfer the recordings to the articulator which is then programmed to follow the tracings. Recently a computerised system has been developed which eliminates the transfer (Denar Pantronic).

Stereographs   Clutches are made to fit the teeth and the patient performs lateral and protrusive excursions. Cutting studs in one clutch cut into the opposing clutch (fig. 5.23). By transferring the clutches to the articulator, and allowing it to move along paths determined by the cut out areas, the condyles can mould cold cure resin placed in the articulator fossae to reproduce the original jaw movements.

Conclusion

The purpose of this chapter has been to describe briefly the several types of articulator and the principal uses of such instruments. Techniques for recording the retruded axis position have been described, and are essential for diagnosis. The facebow device has briefly been discussed together with

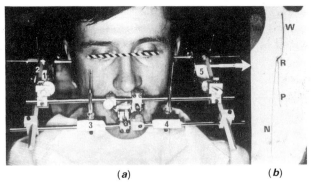

(a)   (b)

Fig. 5.22(a) Stuart pantograph assembled on patient. Tracing plates 1 to 6 are shown. (b) One tracing plate showing (R) the retruded position (N) non-working side movement, (W) working side movement, (P) protrusive movement. The pantograph is reassembled on the articulator. The condylar controls are adjusted until the articulator movement allows the styli of the pantograph to retrace the tracings 1 to 6.

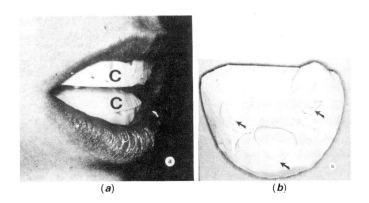

(a)   (b)

Fig. 5.23(a) Clutches (C) from the TMJ system. Cutting studs in the upper clutch, cut the lower clutch when the mandible is moved. (b) Stereographic recording used to programme the TMJ articulator. Cutting studs on the opposing clutch have cut pathways (arrowed) in lateral and protrusive movements. The upper and lower clutches are reassembled on the articulator. Acrylic is allowed to cure in the articulator fossae while the clutches are moved over each other, thereby guiding the articulator movement. The condyle balls mould the fossae.

its use, and, for a more detailed description of the instruments available and their uses the reader is referred to Dawson[3] and Celenza.[6] As stated by Dawson, 'the simpler the articulating device, the more compensations must be made for its shortcomings. But if compensations can be made easily and accurately, there is practical value in keeping the instrumentation as simple as possible.'

References

1 Glossary of prosthodontic terms. *J. Prosthet Dent* 1977; **38**: 70–109.
2 Zarb G A, Speck J E. The treatment of mandibular dysfunction. In *Temporomandibular joint function and dysfunction*, Zarb G A, Carlsson G E (ed) pp 378–381. Copenhagen: Monksgaard. 1979.
3 Dawson P E. In *Evaluation, diagnosis and treatment of occlusal problems*, pp 133–135. St Louis: C V Mosby, 1979.
4 Lundeen H, Wirth C G. Condylar movement patterns engraved in plastic blocks. *J Prosthet Dent* 1973; **30**: 866–875.
5 Tupac R G. Clinical importance of voluntary and induced Bennett movement. *J Prosthet Dent* 1978; **40**: 39–43.
6 Celenza F V. An analysis of articulators. *Dent Clin North Am* 1979; **23**: 305–326.

Moyco Dental Wax, Item No 116-56630, Beauty Pink, X Hard: Moyco Industries Inc, Philadelphia, PA 19132, USA; also available through Cottrell and Co, 15 Charlotte Street, London W1.
Dental Foil Gauge No 10: Minerva (Cardiff) Ltd, 13/15 Fitzalan Place, Cardiff. Available through Cottrell & Co, 15 Charlotte Street, London W1.
Grant Water Bath: Grant Instruments (Cambridge) Ltd, Barrington, Cambridge CB2 5QZ; also available from Cottrell and Co, 15 Charlotte Street, London W1.
Kerr's Bite Registration Paste: Kerr Manufacturing Co, 28200 Wick Road, Romulus, Michigan 48174, USA; also available from Cottrell and Co, 15 Charlotte Street, London W1.
Kerr's Temp Bond: Kerr Manufacturing Co, 28200 Wick Road, Romulus, Michigan 48174, USA; also available from Cottrell and Co, 15 Charlotte Street, London W1.
Hydroflask: Hawley Russell, Leighton House, 35 Darkes Lane, Potters Bar, Hertfordshire.
Whipmix Articulator: available through P Clark and Co, 43 Devonshire Street, London W1, and M J Dental Supplies Ltd, 100 High Street, Ramsey, Cambridgeshire PE17 1BS.
Denar Mark II; Denar Pantronic: Denar Corporation, 2020 Howell Avenue, Anaheim, California, USA. Available through Orthomax Ltd, Carr House, Carrbottom Road, Bradford BD5 9B.
Panadent: Panadent Corporation, Colton, California, USA; not Panadent UK.
Denar: Denar Corporation, 2020 Howell Avenue, Anaheim, California, USA. Available through Orthomax Ltd, Carr House, Carrbottom Road, Bradford BD5 9B.

6 Introduction to Occlusal Adjustment and Posterior Restoration

This chapter considers principles of occlusal adjustment and of posterior restorations. Adjustment is a frequent precursor to restoration. The dentist should prescribe the occlusal form of all restorations: the opposing contacts should not occur by chance.

Occlusal adjustment is the process in which the occlusal surfaces of opposing teeth are altered by the dentist in order to change the relationship of the occlusal contacts. Occlusal adjustment is usually a planned procedure, but may occur unintentionally during tooth preparation (see Chapter 3).

Although the terms are often used synonymously, occlusal adjustment should be differentiated from occlusal equilibration, which is the planned alteration of the occlusal surfaces of teeth to provide stable jaw relationships with stable simultaneous multiple even contacts between opposing teeth. This is usually carried out in two stages, stage 1 being the alteration of occlusal contacts and stage 2 the provision of occlusal stability.

It is frequently easy to alter the occlusion, but subsequently difficult to provide stable tooth-to-tooth contacts. In this chapter, the principles of occlusal adjustment and equilibration will be presented.

Occlusal adjustment can range from adjustment of a single tooth, to adjustment of the entire dentition. When the entire dentition is adjusted, the ultimate aim is one of occlusal equilibration.

Occlusal adjustment

Intercuspal position

In its simplest form occlusal adjustment will consist of alteration of the occlusal surfaces of teeth in the intercuspal position (ICP). Frequently this will be carried out prior to restorative therapy.

In figure 6.1(*a*) the palatal cusp of |7 has over-erupted into the scooped out amalgam |7. In the right lateral excursion (figs. 6.1(*b*) and (*c*)) the over-erupted palatal cusp of |7 was a non-working side contact against the weakened buccal wall of |7 (weakened through previous caries and placement of restorations), and the latter fractured. Replacement of the amalgam should be preceded by shortening of the palatal cusp of the |7 (fig. 6.2(*a*)) and subsequent placement of the opposing restoration to the correct occlusal form (fig. 6.2(*b*)). In lateral excursion the palatal cusp of |7 will now be clear of the buccal cusp of the |7 reducing the risk of fracture (fig. 6.2(*c*)). Such an adjustment is in the intercuspal position, although lateral excursions are obviously observed.

The presence of a plunger cusp (fig. 6.3) requires occlusal adjustment so as to prevent food packing.

Retruded contact position

It is possible to adjust the cuspal inclines in the retruded contact position (RCP) such that when the masticatory muscles contract there is neither an anterior component of force directing the mandible forwards into the intercuspal position, nor a lateral component directing it sideways (fig. 6.4).

The sagittal plane

Large vertical with small horizontal discrepancy between RCP and ICP
In such situations when the initial contacts are removed in the retruded

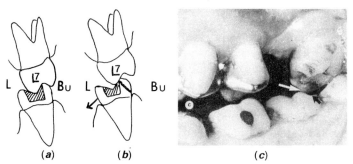

(*a*)   (*b*)   (*c*)

Fig. 6.1 Buccolingual diagram (Bu=buccal, L=lingual) through |7 |7. (*a*) Intercuspal position. The palatal cusp of |7 has over-erupted into the 'scooped out' amalgam of |7. (*b*) The palatal cusp of |7 and buccal cusp of |7 form a non-working side contact in right lateral excursion, leading to fracture of the |7 buccal wall. (*c*) Over-erupted |7 mesio-palatal cusp and fractured disto-buccal cusp of |7, right lateral excursion. |7 |7 are non-working side contacts.

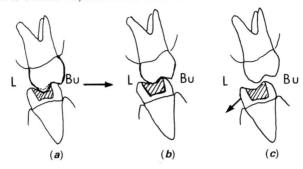

(a)   (b)   (c)

Fig. 6.2 Buccolingual diagrams (Bu=buccal, L=lingual) through |7 |7̄. (*a*) Prior to restoration of |7̄ the palatal cusp of |7 should be reshaped. Shortening the cusp is shown dashed. (*b*) The fossa of the restoration is built up so as to contact the opposing cusp in the ICP. (*c*) In right lateral excursion the anterior guidance separates the now shorter palatal cusp of |7 from |7̄, yet a stabilising contact remains in the ICP.

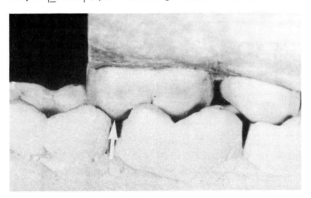

Fig. 6.3 Plunger cusp. Lingual view of the palatal cusp of |6 which wedges between |6̄7̄ resulting in food packing.

contact position, the consequent change in vertical dimension (fig. 6.5) results in an adjusted position being almost coincident with the original intercuspal position, particularly if the adjustment is continued to slight overclosure. There is very little adaptation required by the patient and such an adjustment is easy to carry out and predictable in its results, especially if there is no lateral component to the RCP–ICP discrepancy. The occlusal adjustment technique described by Schluger *et al.*[1] is applicable to this type of RCP–ICP discrepancy. Those interested are also recommended to read Dawson[2] who provides an excellent description of cusp warping to achieve stability. It must be emphasised that for the RCP–ICP discrepancy

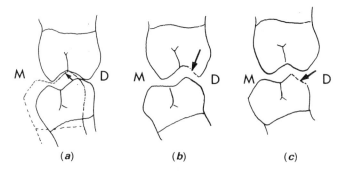

Fig. 6.4 Sagittal plane diagram (M=mesial, D=distal), for example between the disto-buccal cusp of tilted ⌐6 and disto-palatal cusp of |6. (*a*) Contact in the RCP (*solid outline*). If the patient squeezes, the mandible is forced forwards by the action of the cusp inclines, resulting in the ICP (*dashed*). (*b*) Adjustment of the upper cusps can eliminate the inclined plane action (*arrow to broken line*) and/or (*c*) Adjustment of the lower cusp can eliminate the inclined plane action (*arrow to broken line*).

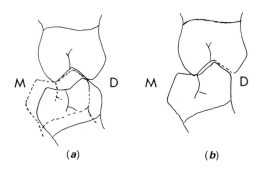

Fig. 6.5 Sagittal plane diagram (M=mesial, D=distal). (*a*) Large vertical with small horizontal dimension between RCP (*solid*) and ICP (*broken*). (*b*) Removal of deflective contacts (*broken line*) leading to altered vertical dimension in the RCP with arcing of the mandible. RCP and original ICP are almost coincident.

described little difference remains between the two positions at the end of adjustment.

Large horizontal with small vertical discrepancy between RCP and ICP
Following adjustments in the retruded contact position, the mandible will frequently reposition itself further distally from the original intercuspal position, resulting in a large horizontal table between the retruded contact position and the original intercuspal position (fig. 6.6) a long centric. It may be difficult for the patient to accommodate to such a long centric if it is

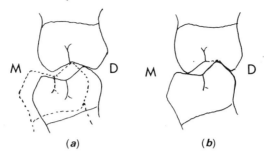

(a) (b)

Fig. 6.6 Sagittal plane diagram (M=mesial, D=distal). (*a*) Large horizontal with small vertical dimension between the RCP (*solid*) and ICP (*broken*). Removal of deflective contacts with little change of vertical dimension in the RCP. There is little arcing of the mandible so that the adjusted RCP is distal to the original ICP.

greater than 1·0 mm, and the multiple tooth-to-tooth contacts that will occur in protrusive and lateral excursions may result in a squeaking sound.

Intermediate group
It is difficult to fit some patients into the previous categories. However, in the absence of a well-defined large vertical and small horizontal component it should be assumed that following occlusal adjustment an area of freedom will remain, frequently being less than 1 mm. Many authors recommend that all patients be provided with such an area.[3] The principles described by Dawson[2] and the technique of Ramfjord and Ash[4] are recommended for the large horizontal and intermediate types of discrepancy. However, when indicated adjustment as in the first type is easy and predictable.

The frontal plane
The presence of a lateral slide can be determined by observing the 1|1 1̅|1̅ centre lines during the movement from the RCP–ICP (fig. 4.5). If present such a slide can be eliminated by adjustment of the appropriate cusps. For example, if the slide is to the left with initial contact on the left, adjust either the buccally facing inclines of upper teeth and/or the lingually facing inclines of the lower teeth on this side (fig. 6.7(*a*)). If the contacts are on the left side with a slide to the right (fig. 6.7(*b*)) the palatally facing inclines of upper teeth and/or buccally facing inclines of lower teeth will be adjusted. The principles described by Dawson[2] should be understood before attempting such an adjustment.

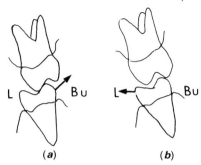

(a)   (b)

Fig. 6.7 Buccolingual diagram through |6 |6̄ (Bu=buccal, L=lingual). (*a*) Initial contact in the RCP. The inclined plane action would force the mandible to the patient's left (*arrow*). Adjustment is to buccally facing inclines of upper teeth and/or lingually facing inclines of the lowers. (*b*) If the initial RCP contact is on the left and results in a slide to the patient's right, then the palatally facing inclines of the upper teeth and/or buccally facing inclines of the lowers are adjusted.

Lateral excursions

Working side contacts   It is possible by occlusal adjustment to alter the tooth surfaces which contact during lateral excursion (fig. 6.8). It can be seen that by altering the lingual incline of an upper tooth the guidance has been changed. Regardless of the tooth or teeth that guide the movement in lateral excursion, the movement should be smooth and result in minimal deflection of the guide tooth in a buccolingual plane. Lateral guidance can be from a single canine (canine guidance), several teeth (group function), or all the teeth on the working side (group function). Adjustment is frequently simplified if the guidance is towards the front of the mouth, that is on the canines.

Non-working side contacts   It is often possible to eliminate contact on the non-working side by occlusal adjustment. Restorations should never introduce non-working side contacts and teeth requiring occlusal restorations should be adjusted accordingly to remove such contacts prior to preparation (fig. 6.9).

Protrusive adjustment
It is frequently difficult to adjust an occlusion to provide simultaneous multiple anterior protrusive contacts, without mutilating aesthetics. However, within the confines of clinical sense the aim should be for: all posterior

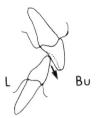

Fig. 6.8 Buccolingual diagram through |3 |3 (Bu=buccal, L=lingual). Adjustment of the palatal incline of the upper canine (*broken line*) will result in an altered lateral guidance.

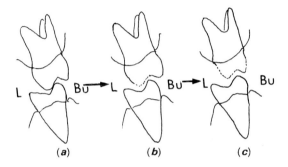

Fig. 6.9 Bucco lingual diagram (Bu=buccal, L=lingual). Adjustment of non-working side contacts prior to tooth preparation. (*a*) |6 to be restored, but it has a non-working side contact with |6. (*b*) Adjust contact before preparation. (*c*) Prepare the tooth with even reduction. There will now be sufficient room for the restorative material without reintroducing the non-working side contact. (See fig. 3.5.)

contacts to be eliminated except in the so-called Class III cases where this is not feasible; movement to be smooth with minimal deflection of anterior teeth; in straight protrusion 'the lower incisors should contact the two upper central incisors from the moment of initial contact in protrusive out to and including the matching incisal edge contacts; in lateral protrusion the lower incisors and canines should contact the upper central, lateral and canine and at no time contact only the upper lateral incisor. These contacts are also in group relationship from their initial contact out to and including their matching edges' (quoted from Anderson *et al.*[5]).

'Crossover'
As the mandibular teeth move past the canines in their lateral and latero-protrusive excursions, the anteriors should remain in contact on their

incial edges and not be separated by any posterior tooth contacts on either the working or non-working sides.[5]

Equilibration

Frequently occlusal adjustment to eliminate deflective contacts should progress to equilibration, which implies that in the RCP (and ICP if not coincident) there will be simultaneous multiple even tooth-to-tooth contacts directed through the long axes of all posterior teeth. There will not be a slide between RCP and ICP when muscle force is applied in RCP. In lateral excursions there will be smooth guidance from the working side with absence of non-working side contacts and in protrusion there will be absence of posterior contacts. The equilibration should result in stable tooth and jaw relationships.

Stability

Most authors agree that to achieve stability following occlusal equilibration cusps must not contact single inclined planes in the RCP or ICP; there must not be a slide between RCP and ICP, either anterior or lateral; occlusal loads should be directed through the long axes of teeth with cuspal contacts located towards the centres of the opposing fossae. Particularly in the case of unsplinted units, tooth positions should be maintained by sound interproximal contacts and opposing contact relations such as cusp tip to fossa contacts, tripod contact, or cusp to marginal ridge contact.

Cusp to fossa contacts
The type of cusp to fossa contact provided will vary depending on the tooth relationships. The simplest arrangement is:

(1) *Cusp tip to fossa (fig. 6.10), no lateral contacts*   In this the opposing cusp tip is arranged to fit into the fossa and lateral excursions are cleared so that the cusp tip only contacts in the RCP–ICP position and immediately discludes in all excursions.

(2) *Cusp to fossa and working side contacts*   Similar to (1), but working side contacts are provided on the lingual incline of the upper buccal cusp against the buccal incline of the lower buccal cusp.

(3) *Tripodism*   Three points of contact are arranged around the convexly shaped sides of the cusp (fig. 6.11(*a*)). This is difficult to achieve in occlusal adjustment and on plastic restorations. The advantage of this type of arrangement is that it theoretically enables greater stability to be achieved

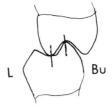

6.10 Buccolingual diagram (Bu=buccal, L=lingual). Cusp tip to fossa contacts.

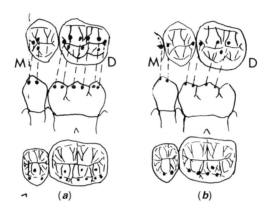

6.11 Mesiodistal diagrams (M=mesial, D=distal). Top=occlusal view of |56. Centre=buccal view of |56. Lower=occlusal view of |56. (*a*) Tripodism: 3 points of contact arranged around the tip of the lower buccal cusps, contact 3 points in the upper fossae. Similar contacts are arranged around the palatal cusps to contact with the lower fossae. (*b*) Cusp marginal ridge contacts.

by providing three repositioning forces without the dangers of rubbing contacts.

Cusp to marginal ridge contacts
Frequently contacts must be arranged between cusps and opposing marginal ridges. However, this can usually be combined with a cusp fossa contact for additional stability (fig. 6.11(*b*)).

No studies are available which either report greater stability of one type of occlusal scheme relative to another, or enable the clinician to determine which teeth are likely to be unstable unless corrected. There are however, some clinical guides:

(1) The degree and type of stabilisation required from opposing contacts

depend upon whether the teeth are individual units or splinted; there is increased mobility and/or reduced bony support; the arch is intact; the teeth are tilted.

(2) Equilibration cannot always achieve stability. Restoration is sometimes required.

(3) Diagnosis should usually include adjustment of mounted casts (always for the neophyte).

(4) Learn how to adjust by starting on teeth that will be prepared for restoration. In this way the subsequent preparation will remove any learning error.

(5) Large vertical/small horizontal cases are easier than large horizontal/small vertical cases so start with the former type.

Posterior restorations

Regardless of the type or number of restorations, the overall aims are similar:

(1) Tooth-to-tooth stability following restoration: the arrangement should be as in figure 6.12(a), not as in figure 6.12(b) in which instability can occur with tilting of teeth.

(2) The restoration must not introduce deflective contacts.

(3) Simultaneous contact of restoration and other teeth in the ICP, that is no high spots and no infra occlusion.

(4) Absence of non-working side contacts on the restoration.

(5) Absence of working side interference on the restoration.

(6) Anterior guidance not interference (see Chapter 9).

(7) Direction of forces through the strongest areas of restorative material and tooth (fig. 6.13).

(8) Direction of forces through the long axes of teeth.

Regardless of the number or type of restorations, there are essentially two occlusal approaches to restorative therapy: the conformative and the reorganised.

The conformative approach

Restorations are provided in harmony with the existing jaw relationships.[6] The intercuspal position should be maintained.

Two situations arise.

(1) The occlusion is untouched prior to tooth preparation, although small changes may then be made on the restorations, such as elmination of the non-working (rubbing) contacts on an amalgam (fig. 6.14).

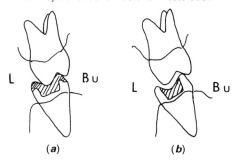

(a)   (b)

Fig. 6.12 Buccolingual diagram (Bu=buccal, L=lingual). (a) Stable relationship between a restoration and the opposing tooth. Compare this with (b) where the relationship is unstable.

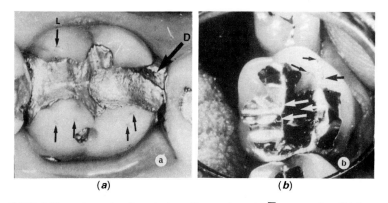

(a)   (b)

Fig. 6.13(a) The only occlusal contact on the amalgam in ⎡7 was on the distal marginal ridge D. This compounded other obvious clinical errors, such as poor cavity design leading to fracture. Other contacts are arrowed, and note the lingual contact L. This is liable to result in fracture of the weakened mesio-lingual cusp. (*occlusal contacts arrowed*) (b) In another tooth, occlusal loads are directed through the strongest parts of the restoration and remaining tooth. Compare this to (a).

(2) The occlusion is modified by localised occlusal adjustment before tooth preparation, that is shortening of an opposing cusp, elimination of non-working side interferences, and removal of a deflective contact on the tooth to be restored (fig. 6.15).

The reorganised approach
The entire occlusal scheme is modified and restoration provided in harmony with new jaw relationships (fig. 6.16) so as to:

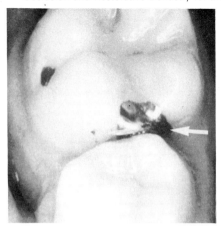

Fig. 6.14 Minimal amalgam. The cavity preparation was minimal so that the amalgam fits in with the existing occlusion, that is it conforms.

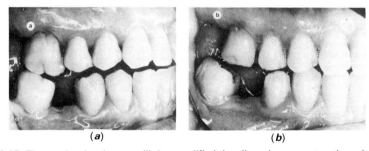

(a)   (b)

Fig. 6.15 The occlusal scheme will be modified locally prior to restoration. (a) 6͞| over-erupted and forms a non-working side contact with 7͞|. (b) 6͞| shortened before 75͞| were prepared for the bridge.

(1) Provide a reproducible starting point, that is the retruded position, particularly when full mouth restoration is required.

(2) Provide an even, stable occlusion.

(3) Provide an occlusion that is in harmony with border movements.

(4) Ensure that iatrogenic deflective contacts are not introduced.

(5) Overcome the inadequacies of restorative materials available today, that is, differential wear and wear which does not match the natural wear of the dentition, by improving the dentist's and technician's control over opposing tooth contacts.

(6) Provide posterior stability to prevent anterior drifting.

The type of occlusion to be provided is dependent upon:

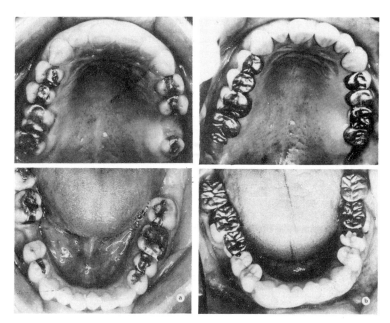

Fig. 6.16 The entire occlusal scheme has been reorganised. (*left, top and bottom*) Before restoration (3 years of drinking 2 bottles of lemonade per day). (*right, top and bottom*) After restoration (large buccal composite restorations necessitated full coverage of 54| 54̅| |45 |4̅5̅).

   (i) The dentist's knowledge, skill and training.

   (ii) The technical assistance that the dentist can receive.

   (iii) The number of restorations required.

   (iv) The presence or absence of a slide from RCP to ICP.

   (v) The dimensions of the RCP/ICP discrepancy if present, that is, large vertical, small horizontal or vice versa.

   (vi) Whether or not the tooth or teeth to be prepared is an initial contact in RCP.

   (vii) Whether or not the restoration is bounded by teeth on each side, or is at the end of the arch (see Chapter 7).

   (viii) Whether or not anterior drifting is present.

   (ix) Whether or not other signs and symptoms of occlusal disturbance are present and to what degree.

Equipment

With cast restorations, articulators are required during fabrication, and these instruments should be used to help achieve the desired result: they are a means to an end, not an end to a means. The technique chosen should be the one that is most suited to the particular restorations. If a compromise is required, it should be determined from knowledge rather than ignorance.

Plastic restorations

Posterior plastic restorations are considered here, while in Chapters 7 and 8 posterior cast and porcelain restorations will be considered.

Single restoration

A small restoration (fig. 6.14) will be restored in a conformative manner, that is, to fit in with the existing jaw relationships, while with a large restoration the opposing cusp should be checked to ensure that it has not over-erupted as a result of wear in the old restoration. If it has, adjustment of the cusp should be carried out prior to renewal of the restoration (fig. 6.2). Following adjustment of the cusp, check it is not a non-working side contact in lateral excursion. Furthermore, during adjustment of the cusp do not grind it horizontally as in figure 6.17(b), but remove either palatal or buccal aspects to try and move the tip of the cusp into the fossa of the opposing tooth (fig. 6.17c). As a general rule a few large restorations will be restored as a conformative occlusion, but localised adjustments should be carried out prior to placement of the restoration.

The relatively poor abrasion resistance of composite restorations limits their use to small occlusal cavities and never large or Class II type restorations.

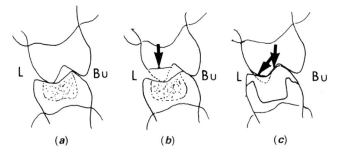

Fig. 6.17 Buccolingual diagram (Bu=buccal, L=lingual). (*a*) The over-erupted cusp of |6 requires adjustment prior to restoration of the opposing |6. (*b*) Do not grind horizontally (*arrow*), this broadens the cusp. (*c*) Grind so as to narrow the cusp (*arrow*) and move the tip into the opposing fossa. Broken line indicates original shape of cusp. |6 restored with an onlay.

Multiple restorations

If large, multiple restorations can constitute an occlusal reconstruction in plastic restorative material. The decision to be made is whether to restore to the existing jaw relationships (conformative occlusion), or to adjust the entire occlusion prior to restoration (reorganised occlusion).

The conformative approach

The amalgams should be placed so as to maintain the existing intercuspal position following preparation of any tooth, that is, complete quadrants should not be prepared at the same time. Preferably alternate teeth should be restored to maintain the original intercuspal position. Retruded or non-working side contacts should not be introduced in the restoration. A decision to work to the existing jaw relationships (or close to them) should be associated with a plan of treatment which will facilitate this.

Indications for conformative placement of multiple amalgams without prior modification of the occlusion are:

(1) Inexperience of the dentist in occlusal adjustment.
(2) Multiple small occlusal restorations.
(3) Coincidence of the retruded contact position with the intercuspal position.
(4) Forward slide RCP to ICP straight and less than 1 mm, patient symptom-free.
(5) Absence of over-erupted cusp into worn or scooped out restoration.

Indications for localised modification of the occlusion prior to placement of multiple amalgam restorations are:

(1) Over-erupted cusps into scooped out amalgams.
(2) Non-working side contacts, particularly if on the teeth to be restored.
(3) Plunger cusps.
(4) Area to be prepared for restoration is a deflective contact on the retruded path of closure. It is prudent in such a situation to adjust this cusp prior to restoration to ensure that mandibular repositioning will not occur during tooth preparation.

The reorganised approach

Frequently, the placement of multiple amalgam restorations constitutes a posterior occlusal reconstruction (fig. 6.18). Unsuspectingly, the dentist may introduce multiple deflective contacts which will lead to subsequent problems (see Chapter 1).

In many circumstances, occlusal 'control and predictability' can be best obtained by occlusal equilibration prior to placement of the amalgams.

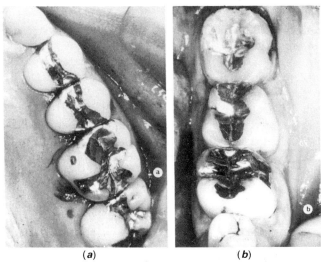

(a)   (b)

Fig. 6.18 One side of the arch reconstructed in amalgam.   (a) Upper left quadrant.
(b) Lower left quadrant.

The indications for a reorganised approach are:

(1) Multiple large restorations required in posterior quadrants.
(2) Slide from RCP to ICP forwards and to one side.
(3) Drifting of anterior segment—this may require posterior occlusal adjustment and retraction of anterior teeth prior to posterior restoration.
(4) Large vertical with small horizontal discrepancy from RCP to ICP. Since such an adjustment is easy to carry out and predictable, it is frequently performed by the experienced operator prior to placement of multiple restorations. It gives him the ability to manipulate the mandible easily, and thereby arrange occlusal contacts in the areas of tooth or restoration which are best able to receive the occlusal loads.

Inexperience of the dentist in occlusal adjustment and equilibration is a definite contra-indication to total mouth adjustment prior to provision of restorations.

By implication it is necessary for the dentist to check the occlusal contacts on the restorations. If the amalgam used does not have a high initial compressive and tensile strengths, then there will be a tendency to place all amalgams out of contact for fear of fracture when testing the occlusion. Therefore the dentist who is concerned about occlusal contacts is committed to using an alloy with a high initial strength, such as the newer spherical or dispersal alloys. This will allow him to check the occlusion and make occlusal adjustments as necessary without fear of fracture. Actual contacts can be located with a shimstock and observed with occlusal indicating tape (fig. 6.19).

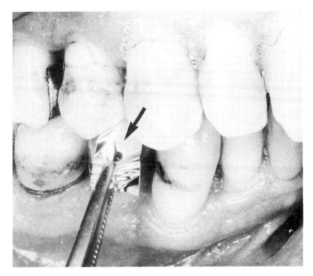

Fig. 6.19 Location of occlusal contacts with shimstock. Resistance to withdrawal indicates occlusal contact.

Conclusion

Several different approaches to occlusal adjustment have been described in the literature. The principles outlined here are common to most of them. The general practitioner should look carefully at his amalgam restorations and provide purposeful occlusal surfaces rather than scooped-out masses of amalgam: posterior occlusal composite restorations are contra-indicated, except for very small Class I restorations.

In Chapters 7 and 8 the approach to posterior cast and porcelain restorations will be described.

References

1 Schluger S, Yuodelis R A, Page R C. *Periodontal disease, basic phenomena, clinical management and occlusal and restorative inter-relationships.* pp 392–400. Philadelphia: Lea and Febiger, 1977.
2 Dawson P E. *Evaluation, diagnosis and treatment of occlusal problems.* pp 80–99. St Louis: C V Mosby, 1974.

3 Tanner H, Ingraham R, and Lundquist D O. The report on the intercuspal position. In: *Occlusion, the state of the art.* Celenza F V, Nasedkin J N. (ed) pp 148–149. Chicago: Quintessence, 1978.

4 Ramfjord S P, Ash M M. *Occlusion.* 2nd ed, pp 271–312. Philadelphia: W B Saunders, 1971.

5 Anderson J A, Isaacson D, O'Bannon J, Wipf H. Consolidated committee report on eccentric relationships. In: *Occlusion, the state of the art.* Celenza F V, Nasedkin J N. (ed) pp 142–145. Chicago: Quintessence, 1978.

6 Celenza F V, Litvak H. Occlusal management in conformative dentistry. *J Prosthet Dent* 1976; **36**: 164–170.

7 Cast Gold and Porcelain Posterior Restorations

When restoring posterior teeth with cast or porcelain restorations, the following points should be considered:
(1) Whether the occlusion should be adjusted prior to placement of a restoration (see Chapter 6).
(2) The type of jaw registration to be used (see Chapter 5).
(3) Whether any check of the accuracy of the registration should be made (see below).
(4) The type of articulator required for the restoration (see Chapter 5).
(5) The occlusal form and contacts (see below).

Assessing jaw registrations

If multiple restorations are to be fabricated in the laboratory, it is reassuring to both the dentist and technician that a system for checking the accuracy of the jaw registration is provided when mounting the casts in an articulator. Reproducibility of several registrations can give the dentist and technician confidence that accurate casts are being used, that a mounting error, such as cast movement has not been introduced in the mounting procedure, that the patient's condyles have not shifted within the fossae between registrations, and that distortion of the occlusal record has not occurred from its registration to the moment of mounting of the cast.

Three useful methods for checking such registrations are the use of a shimstock, the split cast technique, and occlusal copings.

Shimstock
A shimstock is placed between several teeth in the patient's mouth and the

opposing contacts which hold the shimstock are noted (fig. 7.1). The same contacts are subsequently tested on the mounted casts.

Split cast technique[1]

The base of the upper cast is made in two parts: a primary part with deep V-shaped grooves, and a secondary part which fits into these grooves (fig. 7.2(a)) and is attached to the articulator when the upper cast is mounted with a facebow.

Three jaw registrations are taken on the retruded arc of movement, and using one registration, the lower cast is attached to the articulator via the mounted upper cast (fig. 7.2(b)). The registration is then removed, the second registration placed on the occlusal surfaces of the lower cast, and the upper cast separated from its secondary part and seated in this registration (fig. 7.2(c)). The upper member of the articulator is then closed onto the upper cast, and only if the first and second registrations are identical will the split segments meet accurately. It has been demonstrated[1] that a 0·001 inch discrepancy (25·4 μm) between records will result in failure of mating of the split system.

If the second registration fails to match the first registration, the third should be tried and compared. Two registrations should 'check out' before a record is considered to be usable. However, it must be emphasised that this merely demonstrates that the same jaw position has been recorded twice, not necessarily the correct one.

It has been demonstrated recently that for accurate use the split cast system requires a kinematic facebow transfer, unless all jaw registrations are taken at exactly the same vertical dimension, in which case an arbitrary facebow can be used.[2]

Occlusal copings

This technique is particularly suitable when right and left quadrants have

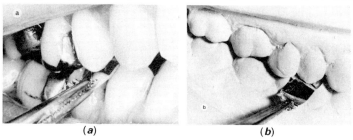

(a)   *(b)*

Fig. 7.1(a) Testing contacts with shimstock in the mouth (test several teeth). **(b)** Testing the same contacts on the mounted casts. Failure to hold indicates errors.

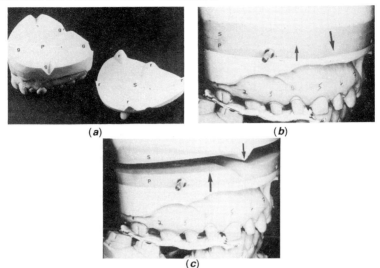

(a)   (b)

(c)

7.2 Split cast system. (*a*) Primary cast P with deep V-shaped grooves g (this is the base of the upper cast.) Secondary cast S with ridges r that fit the grooves. It is attached to articulator. (*b*) Cast mounted via jaw registration, split cast is not separated (*arrows*). (*c*) Split cast separated (*arrows*). Upper cast placed in new registration and upper member of the articulator closed. (With Arcon Articulator remember to hold the fossae against the condyles.) If the registrations in (*a*) and (*b*) are identical, the split casts will mate.

been prepared for restoration. The working casts are mounted in an articulator and small plastic copings (such as Duralay) made on four prepared teeth, one posterior and one anterior on each side (unless the anteriors are in contact, in which case a coping on the last teeth left and right is sufficient). To avoid damage, it is important not to use master dies to make the copings. The copings are built up so as to contact the opposing tooth using a bead-on technique (fig. 7.3). The contact is checked with a shimstock (fig. 7.4(*a*)), then the copings are placed on the teeth (in the mouth) and checked for contact with a shimstock (fig. 7.4(*b*)).

If the shimstock slips easily between the copings and the opposing tooth, it indicates a discrepancy between the mounted casts and the actual contacts in the mouth.

In summary, the stages for checking the coping technique are:

(1) Prepare the teeth.

(2) Make the jaw registrations.

(3) Mount the casts in the dental articulator.

(4) Apply a separating medium (cold mould seal) to spare dies of the preparations.

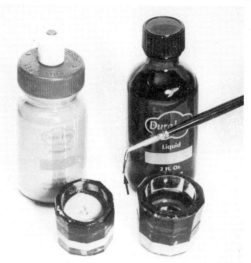

Fig. 7.3 Bead-on technique. One dappens dish contains polymer and one contains monomer. Dip an OO brush into the monomer and then touch it in the polymer powder (middle not edge) to pick up a bead (*arrowed*). Add the bead to the coping. Clean the brush in fresh monomer.

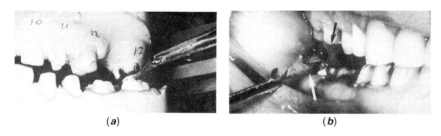

(a)   (b)

Fig 7.4(a) Working casts have been mounted and plastic copings built to contact the opposing teeth on both sides of the arch. Shimstock is used to check contacts. (**b**) The copings have been transferred to the mouth and contacts are checked with shimstock. They should be identical to those on the mounted casts ((**b**) is opposite side to (**a**) and anterior teeth contact therefore anterior copings are not required).

(5) Make the plastic copings over the preparations (Duralay), preferably on a second or duplicate cast (one anterior and one posterior tooth on each side unless the anterior teeth are in contact, in which case distal copings are sufficient but check the shimstock between the copings and between anteriors).

(6) Build up the copings to contact the opposing preparation or tooth (fig. 7.4(*a*)).
(7) When set, check holding with the shimstock.
(8) Transfer the copings to the mouth.
(9) Ask the patient to close and check the shimstock can be held (fig. 7.4(*b*)).

Aims of restored occlusal form

Various theories have been proposed to define the ideal form of the restored occlusal surface. The aims have been listed in Chapter 6. The consensus appears to be that where possible cusps should fit into opposing fossae in the intercuspal position and, where applicable, the retruded position.[3,4] Frequently cusps will have to be warped so as to obtain cusp to fossa relationships, and this can usually only be provided when restoring several contacting teeth and the teeth opposing them. If this cannot be achieved sensibly, cusp marginal ridge contacts should be provided. This will usually occur when individual teeth are restored (fig. 6.11).

In lateral excursions most clinicians would aim to achieve immediate disclusion on the non-working side and either canine guidance or group function on the working side (figs. 7.5(*a*) and (*b*)). In protrusion the aim would be for immediate disclusion anterior to the intercuspal position.

Cusp contact in the intercuspal position

The various cusps have been designated as functional and non-functional.[5] Functional cusps (palatal upper, buccal lower, except for cross-bites) fit into opposing fossae or against marginal ridges and support the vertical dimension in occlusion. Non-functional cusps (buccal upper, lingual lower) hold food in mastication and form one side of an occlusal fossa (fig. 7.6(*a*)). Either three sides or the tip of the functional cusp should contact the opposing fossa in a cusp fossa occlusion.

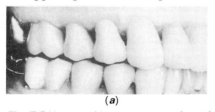 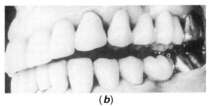

| (*a*) | (*b*) |

Fig. 7.5 Upper and lower reconstruction using bonded porcelain restorations. Right lateral excursion. (*a*) Canine disclusion (The posterior teeth have been designed such that if the canines wear or move group function will result.) (*b*) Note absence of contact on the left, non-working side (distal units on both sides gold not bonded porcelain).

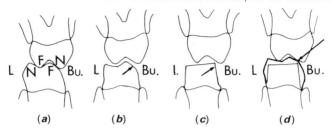

Fig. 7.6 Buccolingual diagram (Bu=buccal, L=lingual) through the first molars to illustrate: (*a*) Functional cusps F, buccal lower, palatal upper and non-functional cusps N, buccal upper, lingual lower. (*b*) Preparation which has a functional cusp bevel (*arrowed*) (*c*) Lack of functional cusp bevel (*arrow*). (*d*) Results in a high crown since the technician requires a minimal thickness for his wax. Perforation will occur during adjustment (*arrow*).

Splinted v unsplinted teeth

The number of occlusal contacts required for stability in splinted units is less than that for unsplinted units. Contacts at the front and the back of the opposing bridges can maintain occlusal stability whereas with single units each tooth requires multiple points of contact to prevent subsequent tipping.

Principles of tooth preparation

If occlusal factors are considered, several basic principles must be applied to tooth preparation:

(1) *Occlusal reduction*   There must be sufficient tooth removal to allow for placement of an adequate bulk of restorative material, 1 mm for gold, 1·5 mm for bonded porcelain.

(2) *Functional cusp bevel*   With a normal buccolingual relationship of opposing teeth, preparations must include a functional cusp bevel: palatal inclines of upper teeth and buccal inclines of lower teeth (fig. 7.6) should allow sufficient room for the restorative material. Failure to do so frequently results in a high restoration, the technician having to bulk out the wax for casting. Subsequent adjustment results in perforation (fig. 7.6). These preparations are fully described by Shillingburg et al.[5]

Waxing

Waxing is best carried out by the wax-added technique. The occlusal form is built up in stages and contacts checked systematically with zinc stearate

Fig. 7.7(a) The wax patterns have been dusted with zinc stearate and contacts appear as black marks (cusp marginal ridge waxing). (*b*) Cusp fossa waxing. (*c*) Castings. (*d*) Upper restorations with sandblasted occlusal surfaces.

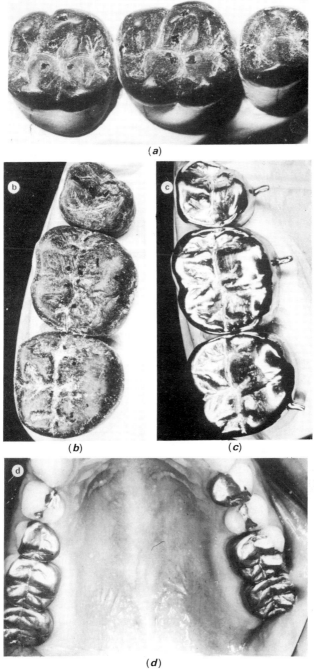

(a)

(b)

(c)

(d)

powder (from any chemist on prescription). The wax is dusted with the powder and opposing casts occluded. Contacts appear as black marks in the white zinc stearate (fig. 7.7). The powder burns out in the furnace. Opposing teeth should be waxed simultaneously. The technique is described in several texts listed in the bibliography p. 186.

Principles applicable to specific gold and porcelain restorations will now be considered.

Single bounded unit (fig. 7.8(a))

Occlusal adjustment

When intact teeth are present on each side of the tooth to be restored the intercuspal position will usually be used (a conformative occlusion) unless there are other cogent reasons for equilibrating the occlusion before restoration. The occlusal adjustment prior to preparation of the teeth would usually be limited to:

(1) The opposing cusp. If the opposing cusp has erupted into a 'scooped out' existing restoration, it is necessary to adjust the opposing cusp before preparation of the tooth to prevent it becoming a non-working side contact later (fig. 6.3). It is better to shorten the opposing cusp and raise the fossa of the restored tooth so as to provide good contact in the intercuspal position and freedom in lateral excursion than to work to the over-erupted tooth and deepen the fossa of the restoration.

(2) Initial contact in the retruded position of the tooth to be prepared. For reasons given in Chapter 4 (Retruded Contact Position) it would be necessary to adjust or remove this contact to avoid any unwanted consequences.

Record type

The intercuspal position should be recorded. Frequently the casts may be manually positioned and no registration is necessary. Occasionally, if the crown to be replaced is occlusally intact, a plaster index can be made and the new crown made to copy the existing one (fig. 7.8(b)), or a temporary crown made, carefully adjusted and copied. If there is any doubt, however, an intercuspal record must be made with the teeth in contact. The record should only contact the prepared tooth and its opposing number and should not encroach on the occlusal surfaces of adjacent teeth. Three simple methods will be described. In all cases the patient should close but not squeeze, since solid casts will not reproduce the tooth movement that

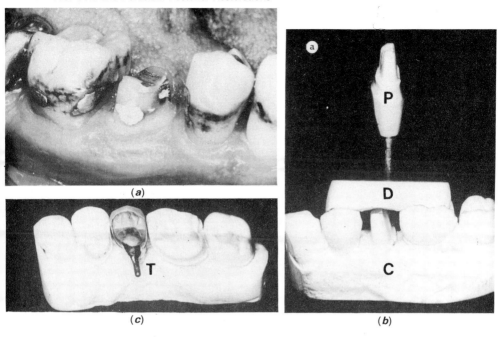

(a)

(c)   (b)

Fig. 7.8(a) Single bounded unit prepared for full crown. The occlusion of existing crown was acceptable. Replacement was necessary because of caries. (*b*) A plaster index was made of the existing occlusal surface intra-orally, to include one tooth mesially and distally. The index p was positioned on a quadrant cast C. (NB solid cast C. Separate die D). This enabled the technician to copy the original form (*c*) Tag T is to assist removal at try-in and is subsequently removed.

may occur. The prepared tooth, being unopposed, would not have the same relationship to the adjacent teeth on the records as on the casts. This is of particular significance with mobile teeth.

Wax

Soft wax cannot be used and a hard wax (Moyco Beautihard) is preferred. The wax is softened at 55°C and a small portion cut to fit between the teeth. It is wrapped around a piece of x-ray lead foil positioned over the prepared tooth and the patient closes into the intercuspal position (fig. 7.9). It is imperative to achieve shallow indentations of the opposing tooth into the wax and it is chilled while *in situ*. Deep indentations make accurate location of the cast difficult. This record must be used quickly, to avoid distortion on storage.

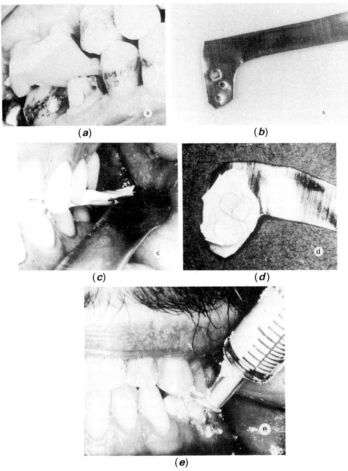

Fig. 7.9 Intercuspal registrations. (*a*) Wax. (*b*) Soft metal cut to shape. (*c*) Soft metal and registration paste in mouth. (*d*) Record removed. (*e*) Bite stone syringed between the preparation and opposing teeth.

Paste

A piece of soft metal is taken and cut as in figure 7.9(*b*). The small extension passes between the prepared tooth and the opposing tooth. Small holes are made in the metal for retention of the bite registration paste. The patient is rehearsed to close into the intercuspal position, and bite registration paste is mixed and placed on both sides of the registration holder. This is placed over the prepared tooth using the extension as a handle and the patient

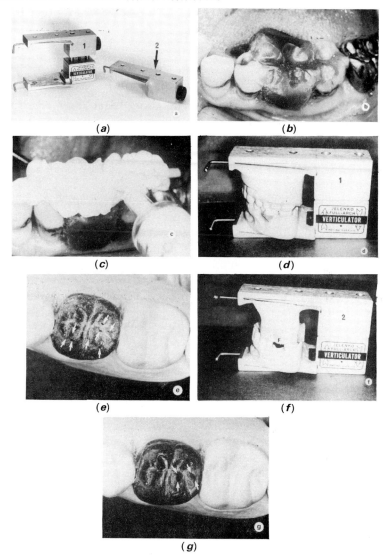

(a)   (b)

(c)   (d)

(e)   (f)

(g)

Fig. 7.10 FGP technique for single unit. (*a*) Verticulator, note the two upper portions 1 and 2. (*b*) Wax in place on preparation and has been contoured by the opposing cusps (Ensure that over-erupted cusps are recontoured prior to making FGP.) (*c*) Bite stone syringed over wax and adjacent teeth. (*d*) Full arch working and opposing casts mounted in the verticulator via an ICP registration. (*e*) ICP contacts on wax (*arrowed*). (*f*) FGP index F positioned on ⌐456 and plastered to verticulator portion 2 and then closed on wax pattern. (*g*) Non-working side contacts (*arrowed*). These must be eliminated leaving only the ICP contacts.

closes into the intercuspal position (fig. 7.9(c)) which is maintained until the medium sets.

Plaster

Bite stone is mixed in a bowl and loaded into a disposable syringe. The patient closes into the intercuspal position and the plaster is syringed between the teeth and the position held until the plaster has set (fig. 7.9(e)). This method has the advantage of ensuring that the patient is in the intercuspal position before any registration medium is used. The disadvantage is that the time of setting is longer than for the other two methods, and the stone can be affected by saliva. Do not use this method for patients with excess salivation.

In the author's opinion the more stable registrations of either bite registration paste or bite stone are to be preferred to the wax method which will frequently distort. Rigid records should only be used if silver plated dies or two stone dies are available, that is the working casts and a separate master die, in case the die is chipped. There are obviously many individual variations which can be made to the above techniques.

It is advisable to observe with a shimstock which teeth contact in the mouth and to note and confirm this on the casts before and after fabricating the restoration.

Equipment

Hand held casts Sometimes single gold restorations can be reasonably fabricated on hand held casts. However, difficulties can occur when refinement of the cuspal contacts is attempted. Porcelain occlusal surfaces are difficult to refine by this method because if high the powder breaks off, particularly when testing lateral excursions.

Plane line articulator The disadvantages of this instrument have been discussed in Chapter 5.

Cast holder and functionally generated path (FGP) technique
A convenient cast holder termed the Verticulator is made for this technique (fig. 7.10(a)). The upper and lower halves are related by guide rods and flat surfaces. Two upper portions are available, one for the opposing cast and one for the FGP. Lateral excursions of the instrument are not required since these are contoured in the FGP. Apposition of the two parts of the instrument maintains the vertical dimension of the ICP.

This technique is suitable for the single restoration. The stages are:

(1) The opposing tooth is observed in lateral excursion and if an interference or an over-erupted cusp is present this is adjusted.

(2) The tooth to be restored is reduced occlusally, and it is confirmed that it is free from the opposing tooth, in all excursions.

(3) Soft wax is applied to occlusal surfaces of the prepared tooth (Bosworth's Tacky Wax is useful for this) and stabilised by moulding it to the interproximal undercuts or attaching it to a compound coping made on the preparation.

(4) The patient grinds in all excursions, so that the opposing tooth cuts pathways into the wax. Ensure that the wax remains stable on the prepared tooth (fig. 7.10(b)).

(5) Check that the wax has been contoured in all excursions (fig. 7.10(b)).

(6) Mix 'Bite stone'.

(7) Load into a disposable syringe.

(8) Syringe stone over the wax and teeth on each side of the prepared tooth (fig. 7.10(c)).

(9) Allow to set.

(10) Remove from mouth and remove the wax from the underside of the stone 'index'.

(11) Complete the preparation of tooth.

(12) Take the impression of the preparation and opposing arch—full arch impressions are necessary for accuracy of mounting.

(13) Intercuspal jaw registration.

(14) Mount the casts in the verticulator (fig. 7.10(d)), or simple hinge articulator.

(15) When using the verticulator, remove the upper member and position the second portion.

(16) Seat the stone FGP index on the working cast and plaster it to verticulator second portion.

(17) Replace the opposing cast.

(18) Wax in the normal fashion using the opposing cast to obtain intercuspal contacts.

(19) Dust zinc stearate onto the occlusal surface of the wax and occlude the casts. Black marks through the zinc stearate indicate cuspal contacts (fig. 7.10(e)).

(20) Once occlusal anatomy is complete check the intercuspal contacts.

(21) Dust the occlusal surface with zinc stearate.

(22) Remove the opposing cast and replace with the FGP. (If a simple hinge is used, place the plaster index over prepared arch obtaining accuracy of seating from adjacent teeth.) Close (fig. 7.10(f)). Any

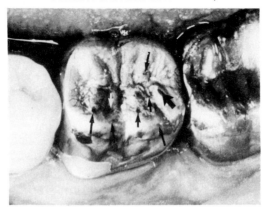

Fig. 7.11 Sandblasted gold occlusal surface showing contacts as shiny areas (*arrowed*).

marks occurring which are excess to the intercuspal position will be working or non-working side contacts in the mouth (fig. 7.10(*g*)).

(23) Eliminate these from carving and refine ICP contacts using the full arch opposing cast.

(24) Cast restoration.

(25) If group function is to be provided, when the functionally generated path index is placed on to the working cast, the contact should be built up on the buccal surface into the index. This will achieve group function in the lateral excursion.

One major failing of the FGP system is that unless the occlusion is initially totally equilibrated, the guidances recorded could be from inclines on other teeth. Subsequent change of the occlusal surfaces of these teeth could alter the functional relationship of restored teeth. Furthermore, mobile teeth will move rather than cut the FGP in the wax. Alternatively, mobile unprepared teeth may move during FGP recording, effectively bringing the prepared tooth closer to the opposing tooth, resulting in a discrepancy between the full arch ICP mounting and the FGP mounting.

Semi-adjustable articulator

Casts can be rapidly mounted without a facebow, using an intercuspal record and average setting for condyles. For most patients the condylar guidance should be set very shallow (approximately 20°) and side shift guides widened (approximately 30°), so that when cusps are built on the restoration and this is transferred back to the mouth, the clearance built into the restoration in lateral and protrusive excursion will be even greater in the mouth (provided the patient has steeper condylar guidance) than on the articulator. Clashing of cusps will therefore be avoided. If non-working contacts are noted on unprepared teeth, these should be slightly relieved on the mounted casts. If the restoration is then made without non-working contacts, it will definitely be clear when returned to the mouth. Do not over reduce unprepared non-working contacts or over flatten the condylar guidance lest the prepared tooth actually contacts its opposing tooth when the articulator is moved.

Checking contacts

The casting should be tried in before cementing with both gold and porcelain restorations. Ensure that the restoration is correctly seated on the preparation before checking the occlusion. Initial contacts on the gold restorations are best detected by sand blasting the occlusal surface with a fine abrasive. They show up as shining areas in the ICP or lateral excursions (fig. 7.11).

Initial contacts on porcelain are more difficult to observe and are best checked either with the thick blue articulating paper (as an initial background) followed by thin occlusal tapes (GHM), or Kerr's occlusal indicator wax placed over the occlusal surface. Perforation of the occlusal indicator wax following closure indicates occlusal contact. Ensure that deflective contacts in the RCP are not introduced by the restoration.

Both types of restoration must be checked to ensure that they are not high and this is done with a shimstock. The shimstock should be held between the restoration and the opposing tooth and between teeth which hold the shimstock when the restorations are not in place. A similar test can be made by the technician on the mounted casts. Adjustments to gold are readily made with white stones in an air rotor handpiece. Porcelain can be adjusted with the Shofu porcelain polishing kit and subsequently polished or preferably reglazed.

Frequently, however, if a restoration is high, the opposing cusp must be shortened, since deepening the fossa on the restoration increases the likelihood of introducing a non-working side contact with the opposing cusp fitting deeper into the restoration.

Single unit at the end of the arch (fig. 7.12)

Occlusal adjustment

This is made as for a bounded unit. If the tooth to be restored is an initial

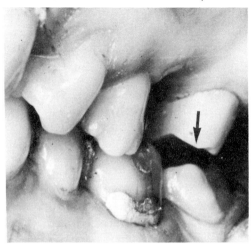

Fig. 7.12 Single tooth prepared at the end of the arch.

contact in the retruded contact position, it must be adjusted prior to restoration (see Chapter 4). Lateral excursion must also be checked and any non-working side contacts eliminated prior to tooth preparation. It can be seen from figure 7.13 that a non-working side contact will probably be re-introduced if it is not eliminated prior to restoration. Any protrusive interferences should similarly be eliminated.

Hand articulation of casts is difficult and a jaw registration in the intercuspal position is required. Similar techniques to those described above can be used. Check with a shimstock as before. Similar articulators to those above are used for the same reasons and similar checks made on cementation.

Fig. 7.13 Buccolingual diagram through three levels. (Bu=buccal, L=patient's left, R=patient's right, Lc=left condyle, F=left fossa). Section through 3| 3|, |7 |7 and the left condyle and fossa.

If a non-working side contact is not eliminated prior to tooth preparation, it is probable that a new non-working contact will be introduced by a restoration. This is due to the reseating of the condyle in the fossa with reduction of interocclusal space. This is particularly liable to occur if the last tooth in the arch is prepared. It is advisable to remove the contact prior to preparation.

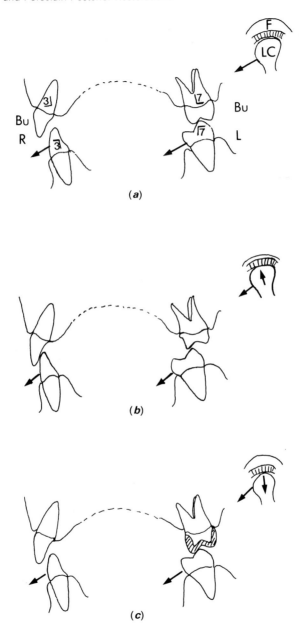

(a)

(b)

(c)

References

1 Lauritzen A G, Wolford L W. Occlusal relationships: the split cast method for articulator techniques. *J Prosthet Dent* 1964; **14**: 256–260.
2 Laing D P, Wise M D. Split cast discrepancies and arbitrary axis dental cast articulator mounting. *J Oral Rehabit* 1978; **5**: 249–259.
3 Schluger S, Yuodelis R A, Page R C. *Periodontal disease, basic phenomena, clinical management and occlusal and restorative inter-relationships.* pp 403, 691. Philadelphia: Lea and Febiger, 1977.
4 Consolidation Committee Reports, In: *Occlusion, the state of the art.* Celenza F V, Nasedking J N. (ed) pp 139–150. Chicago: Quintessence, 1978.
5 Shillingburg H T, Hobo S, Whitsett L D. *Fundamentals of fixed prosthodontics.* p 75. Chicago: Quintessence, 1978.

Duralay Inlay pattern resin: Reliance Dental Manufacturing Co, Worth, Illinois 60482, USA; available through Cottrell & Co, 15 Charlotte Street, London W1.

Moyco Dental Wax, Item No 116-56630, Beauty wax X-hard: Moyco Industries Inc, Philadelphia, PA 19132, USA; available through Cottrell & Co, 15 Charlotte Street, London W1.

Dental Foil gauge No 10: Minerva (Cardiff) Ltd, 13/15 Fitzalan Place, Cardiff; available through Cottrell & Co, 15 Charlotte Street, London W1.

Whip Mix bite stone (white): Whip Mix Corporation, 361 Farmington Avenue, Louisville, Kentucky 40217, USA: available through PMC, 43 Devonshire Street, London W1.

Jelenko Verticulator (full arch): J. F. Jelenko & Co, 170 Petersville Road, New Rochelle, NY 10801, USA; available from Marcel A. Courtin Ltd, Courtin House, Horsham Road, Capel, Surrey.

Bosworth's Tacky Wax: Becker-Parkin Dental, 147 West 42nd Street, New York, NY 10036, USA.

Kerr Occlusal Indicator Wax: Kerr Manufacturing Co, 28200 Wick Road, Romulus, Michigan 48174, USA; available from Cottrell & Co.

Shofu Dura-White stones; Shofu Dental Corp, 4025 Bohannon Drive, Mento Park, California 94925, USA; available from Cottrell & Co.

Shofu Porcelain Polishing Kit: Shofu Dental Corp, 4025 Bohannon Drive, Mento Park, California 94025, USA; available from Cottrell & Co.

---

8 Cast Gold and Porcelain Multiple Posterior Restorations

Three units bounded by teeth on each side (fig. 8.1)

Occlusal adjustment
The same indications for adjustment are present as for the single unit. However, slightly more care must be taken to ensure that the opposing arch has a desirable occlusal plane.

Record type
The intercuspal position is the position of choice and records should be taken by one of the previously described techniques. A further useful technique may be adopted. A cast of the opposing teeth is made and cold mould seal painted on it. Duralay is applied by the bead-on technique (fig. 7.3) to the teeth which will oppose the bridge. The beads are applied to the teeth on the cast and a thin Duralay platform built up. After preparation of the bridge the platform is then taken to the mouth and placed on the teeth and the patient asked to close. Ensure that there is clearance between the platform and the prepared teeth. With the teeth together bite registration paste is inserted between the Duralay platform and the prepared teeth to produce an intercuspal record. If the preparations are non-vital, Duralay can be beaded to the platform and built to touch the prepared teeth (fig. 8.1).

Retruded registration
If there is a history of TMJ dysfunction or bruxism and the dentition has not been adjusted to eliminate retruded deflective contacts, a tooth apart

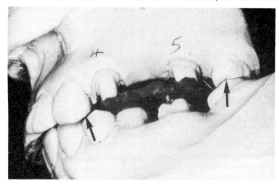

Fig. 8.1 Three units bounded by teeth on each side. A Duralay intercuspal registration is in place.

retruded registration should be made and the cast mounted using this. It is imperative that the articulator chosen for fabrication of the restoration is able to move from the retruded to the intercuspal position, and as such an Arcon type of instrument will be required so that the condyles can come out of the fossae if necessary (fig. 8.2). The restorations are waxed in the intercuspal position, but the use of the retruded mounting will assist in preventing retruded deflective contacts from being introduced on to the bridge work. Adjustment in the mouth will probably be required.

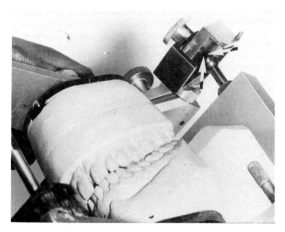

Fig. 8.2 The casts are in the ICP. However, they were mounted with a retruded registration. When the intercuspal position is simulated, the condyles frequently 'separate' from the fossae (*arrows*).

A retruded registration is also made if the occlusion has been equilibrated with or without an area remaining between RCP and ICP. In this situation, however, registration is easier than above since a tooth together registration can be made.

Check with a shimstock as before.

Equipment

The semi-adjustable articulator is the instrument of choice and as stated previously, if the RCP is unadjusted, an Arcon instrument, which allows the condyles to be separated from the fossae, is preferable if a retruded registration is taken. An articulator in which the condyles are fixed in the fossae slot would not allow accurate positioning of the cast in the intercuspal position if only a retruded registration were taken. However, such an instrument can be used with an intercuspal record. Subsequent release of the condyle jack screws will allow the articulator to approximate the RCP. Shallow arbitrary lateral and protrusive settings can be used.

The functionally generated path system described in Chapter 7 can be applied to this situation, provided that the anterior guidance is acceptable (see Chapter 9). Regardless of the method used, all waxing is carried out in the ICP and subsequently checked for lateral, protrusive and retrusive excursions.

Three units at the end of an arch (fig. 8.3)

Occlusal adjustment

Since the occlusal landmarks for virtually one side of the arch will be eliminated during the tooth preparation, it is frequently easier to adjust the entire occlusion (equilibration) prior to tooth preparation. This is es-

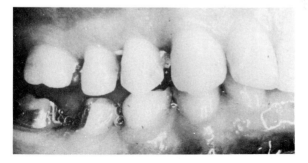

Fig. 8.3 Three units at the end of the arch.

pecially so if the teeth to be prepared are deflective contacts on the retruded arc of closure; and the patient exhibits a large vertical and small horizontal discrepancy between RCP and ICP, since this is easily adjusted.

If the entire occlusion is not adjusted prior to tooth preparation, the approach should be as follows: adjust deflective contacts on the teeth to be prepared, then leave for several weeks to ensure that the patient is comfortable. If not, continue the adjustment until comfortable. Prepare one tooth and make a Duralay coping in the intercuspal position as in figure 8.4. The adjacent teeth can subsequently be prepared and the Duralay coping used to re-establish the intercuspal position so that a conformative occlusion can be provided (that is conforming to the adjusted relationships).

Record type

Preferably the occlusion will have been previously equilibrated and a retruded registration is taken at the correct vertical dimension for restoration, that is with all of the unprepared teeth in contact. If the patient originally had a large vertical and small horizontal discrepancy between RCP and ICP, the retruded position will be virtually coincident with the intercuspal position.

If there remains a long centric (horizontal area between RCP and ICP), it is essential that the articulator used for restoration should be able to move from retruded to intercuspal positions. When semi-adjustable articulators

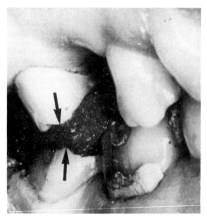

Fig. 8.4 A Duralay coping has been made following preparation of one unit to reposition the mandible in the ICP.

are used, this movement is only approximate and some intra-oral occlusal adjustment should be anticipated.

Check with a shimstock as before, and split casts or copings.

Equipment and methods

A semi-adjustable articulator will usually be used.

Semi-adjustable articulator

Lateral jaw registrations must be taken in order to set the condylar inclinations. These are made with the following equipment: base-plate or Moyco Beauti-pink hard wax, scissors, thermostat-controlled water bath, and soft metal (gauge 10).

The wax is heated to the softening temperature in the water bath and a registration plate made as before. If the casts are already mounted, this wax is placed on the upper cast and the articulator moved to approximately 4 mm of the lateral movement and the lower indentations made. The wax is removed and trimmed with scissors to expose the tips of the buccal cusps of the upper teeth and then re-softened. It is then transferred to the patient's mouth and the patient guided to lateral movement and the indentations refined. It is chilled in the mouth, placed back on the articulator and the opposite condylar inclination and sideshift guide are set, that is, for left lateral movement set the right condylar elements. Details of setting the articulators can be found in Shillingburg *et al.*, or in the instruction manuals for the articulators. Having set condylar inclination and progress-ive sideshift it is advisable to reduce the angle of the condylar guidance by approximately 5° to compensate for the inaccuracies of the semi-adjustable articulator. Cusps waxed on a shallow setting when transferred to the mouth will exhibit greater clearance and give the dentist more flexibility.

Alternatives

A functionally generated path technique can be employed, particularly if equilibration has been carried out. If the FGP system is used ensure that the wax is stable on the preparations. Do not use it if teeth are mobile since the wax will not be properly carved by the opposing teeth or alternatively the guidance teeth may move. Ensure that the anterior guidance is acceptable (see Chapter 9).

Quadrant (fig. 8.5)

The quadrant should be treated similarly to three units at the end of the arch. However, there is more indication for equilibration prior to restoration, and the use of a fully adjustable articulator may be considered.

Fully adjustable articulators require pantographic or stereographic surveys for the programming of lateral excursions and the interested reader is referred to the bibliography.

Two quadrants on opposite sides of the arch or three quadrants (fig. 8.6)

Adjustment
Preferably all cases will be occlusally equilibrated prior to restoration, to eliminate the slide from the retruded to the intercuspal position. Only prepare the teeth when the mandible can be repeatedly manipulated with ease.

Record type
The retruded position is recorded. Lateral and protrusive records must be made, the type depending on the articulator.

Check the jaw registrations by the previously described methods (Chapter 7).

Equipment
Preferably the fully adjustable articulator will be used, but it is feasible to use a semi-adjustable articulator particularly in the following cases:
(1) No symptoms.
(2) Steep anterior guidance, therefore allowing more leeway for arbitrary condylar guidance (fig. 8.7).
(3) Large opposing splinted units, since the need for multiple cusp to fossa contacts is slightly reduced giving more leeway in cusp location. This is not an indication for splinting.
(4) Shallow curve of Spee, since cusps can be made with less fear of clashing.

The indication for the use of a fully adjustable articulator increases if there is a combination of the following:
(1) Previous symptoms.
(2) Shallow anterior guidance, since the leeway for cusp placement is less than with steep guidance (fig. 8.8).

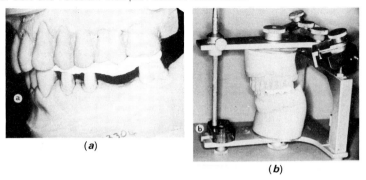

(a)

(b)

Fig. 8.5 The lower left quadrant has been prepared following equilibration. RCP/ICP are coincident. (*a*) Bitestone registration in position. Anteriors in contact. (*b*) Casts mounted in Whipmix articulator. Upper cast previously mounted with facebow.

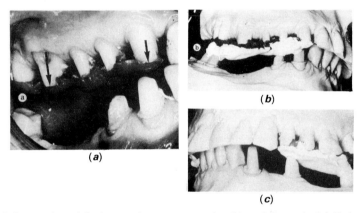

(a)

(b)

(c)

Fig. 8.6 Preparation of 2 plus quadrants on opposite sides of the arch. (*a*) Trying in a Duralay platform made on a spare master cast. (*b*) Temp bond has been added in the mouth to produce a right and left. (*c*) RCP registration.

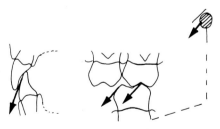

Fig. 8.7 Sagittal plane diagram (condyles shaded, protrusive movement *arrowed*). Steep anterior guidance gives leeway for arbitrary condylar guidance. A semi-adjustable articulator can be used.

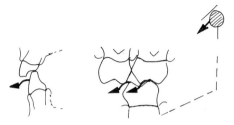

Fig 8.8 Sagittal plane diagram as figure 8.7. Shallow anterior guidance. There is no leeway for arbitrary condylar guidance. If the anterior guidance remains unaltered, a fully adjustable articulator should be used.

(3) Multiple individual units, since it is more important to achieve cusp–fossa contacts for stability.

(4) Steep curve of Spee: short cusps must be used.

(5) Immediate side shift.

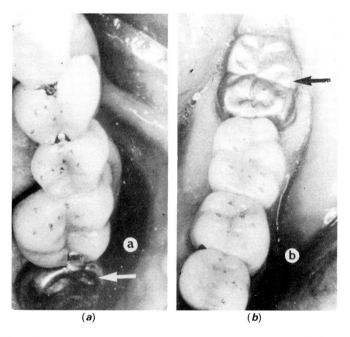

(a)   (b)

Fig. 8.9 Porcelain units opposing each other: (*a*) upper; (*b*) lower. The |7 |7 (*arrowed*) were restored with gold occlusal surfaces to establish an accurate distal occlusal stop. Occlusal contacts are marked.

Porcelain units opposing each other or opposing gold (fig. 8.9)

Often the occlusal aspect of such restorations should be made in metal to achieve optimum contacts. However, this is not always feasible, for aesthetic reasons. Good results for porcelain occlusal surfaces can be achieved by preparing opposing teeth and mounting casts as described previously; waxing the opposing units (fig. 8.10) and then reducing the lower patterns evenly by 1 mm (to allow room for porcelain) and casting. Alternatively, new copings can be made using an index of the lower wax patterns as a guide. The castings are replaced on the mounted cast and porcelain built to the opposing wax patterns, or preferably into the index of the original lower wax patterns. The porcelain is finished, tried in the mouth, stained and glazed. The finished lowers are replaced on the mounted cast (fig. 8.11) and the upper wax patterns refined to them. Contact is provided in the ICP with freedom in excursions. The patterns are cast if gold restorations are required. If porcelain is required a Duralay index is made and attached to the lower member of the articulator (figs 8.12 and 8.13). The upper castings are made with even clearance for the porcelain. The body firing is made just short of the index. The enamel is added to the index and the very thin addition minimises shrinkage[2] (fig. 8.14).

The porcelain is polished and the occlusion checked and adjusted. Following glazing, small additions can be made with low fusing clear porcelain.

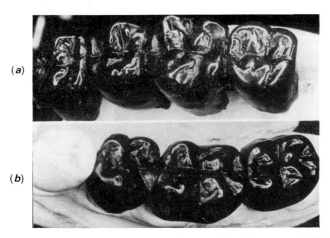

(a)

(b)

Fig. 8.10 Technique for fabricating porcelain occlusals: (*a*) upper and (*b*) lower full wax-ups.

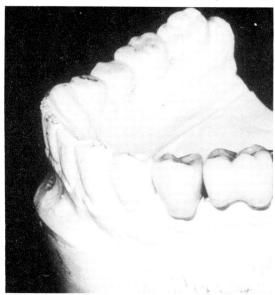

Fig. 8.11 Technique for fabricating porcelain occlusals. $\overline{56}$ returned to articulator after trying in the mouth. ($\overline{7}$ gold and not in place).

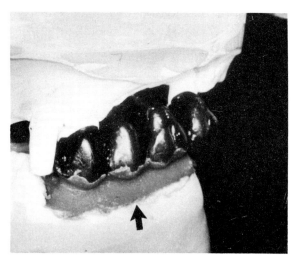

Fig. 8.12 Technique for fabricating porcelain occlusals. Upper wax patterns have been refined to the lower completed units. A Duralay index has been made to the patterns (*arrow*).

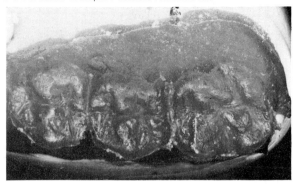

Fig. 8.13 Technique for fabricating porcelain occlusals. Close-up of index.

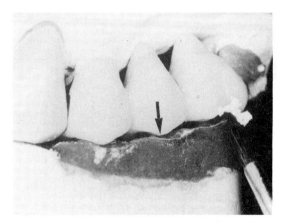

Fig. 8.14 Technique for fabricating porcelain occlusals. Body firing almost to index (*arrow*). Thin enamel layer being added. The thin addition minimises shrinkage.

Conclusion

The basic procedures for various posterior restorations have been outlined and are summarised in Table I (overleaf).

References

1 Shillingburg H T, Hobo S, Whitsett L. D. *Fundamentals of fixed prosthodontics.* pp 223–225. Chicago: Quintessence, 1978.
2 Kuwata M. *Theory and practice for ceramo-metal restorations.* Chicago: Quintessence, 1980.

Table I Summary of procedures for posterior cast gold and porcelain restorations

Type of restoration	Adjust	Record	Check	Equipment
(1) Single bounded unit in gold or porcelain	Opposing cusps plus the tooth to be restored if initial contact in RCP on non-working side contact	Sometimes nil, usually ICP. Sometimes FGP	With shimstock in the mouth and on the casts with and without restorations	Plaster index. Gold, hand held. Porcelain or gold: cast holder plus FGP or semi-adjustable articulator
(2) Single unit at end of arch	If initial contact in RCP. Lateral excursions, particularly non-working and protrusive contacts	ICP. Sometimes FGP	Shimstock	As for porcelain (1)
(3) 3 units bounded	As for single crown but more indication for adjustment	Usually intercuspal. Retruded if instrument allows movement from retruded to intercuspal. Movement will only be an approximation. Lateral wax records or FGP	Shimstock and/or split cast	As above. (Reduce condylar angle 5°)

Table I *continued*

Type of restoration	Adjust	Record	Check	Equipment
(4) 3 units at end of arch	Nearly always local. Entire dentition if deflective contact in RCP, especially if large vertical and small horizontal. Otherwise only the teeth to be prepared	Intercuspal/retruded contact position if adjusted. ICP if unadjusted plus an RCP record to check retruded contacts. Lateral wax records.	Split cast or copings plus shimstock	Semi-adjustable articulator
(5) Quadrant	As for (4) but more indication for equilibration	As for (4)	As for (4)	As for (4) but consider fully adjustable articulator
(6) 2 quadrants on opposite sides, that is both uppers or both lowers, or 3 or more quadrants	Preferably equilibrate, invariably if large vertical and small horizontal RCP–ICP	Retruded position. Lateral wax or pantographic records	Split cast plus copings and shimstock	Preferably fully adjustable but feasible on semi-adjustable if no symptoms, steep anterior guidance, and large splinted units. Fully adjustable articulator required if a combination of shallow anterior guidance, previous symptoms, individual units, steep curve of Spee, and immediate sideshift

9 Restoration of the Anterior Teeth

It is important to understand the effect of contacting surfaces of anterior teeth on mandibular movement (anterior guidance) before restoring anterior teeth (fig. 9.1). Restorations with too shallow an anterior guidance can result in the conflict of opposing posterior cusps and poor aesthetics whereas too steep a guidance can result in increasing mobility or movement of the anterior teeth, mechanical failure of anterior restorations or patient discomfort. At present there are no experimental data available to assist the dentist in his prescription for anterior guidance, but there are certain clinical guidelines.

When restoring anterior teeth, one must decide whether or not to provide near contact between upper and lower incisors and canines in the intercuspal position. Light contact will facilitate anterior guidance whereas spacing between the upper and lower anterior segment makes such guidance difficult to achieve. There are several mechanical advantages in providing anterior guidance for excursive movement:

- It is easier to make adjustments in the front of the mouth than the back.
- Smooth mandibular movement can be produced without posterior teeth jarring.
- Excessive loading of individual teeth can be avoided in excursive movements.
- Stability of anterior teeth can be enhanced by repeated contacts.
- In excursive grinding movements, the mandible, its muscles (especially the masseter) and joints may conveniently be regarded as a third-order lever, therefore for a given effort the force experienced in

147

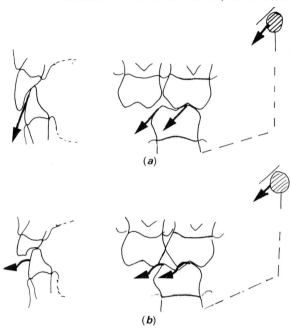

Fig. 9.1 Sagittal plane diagram (*condyles are shaded*) showing protrusive movement (*arrow*). (*a*) Steep anterior guidance. (*b*) Shallow anterior guidance with the same condylar guidance as (*a*) Note the reduced clearance between the posterior teeth during protrusion, leading to clashing of cusps.

the anterior teeth which are furthest away from the fulcrum (TMJ) is less than the posterior teeth. Furthermore, for the same rotation at the condyle, a lower anterior tooth will move further (therefore faster) than a posterior cusp. This is significant in parafunctional activities such as bruxism, since abrasion is directly related to load and inversely related to speed, assuming a standard abrasive.

However, it may not always be possible or desirable to provide anterior guidance. Indeed anterior teeth may remain stable without contacting in the intercuspal position (ICP), being maintained by tongue, lip or occasional 'functional' tooth contacts. Problems may arise when the patient complains of loose or drifting front teeth, when fracture or wear of teeth or restorations occurs, or when the original guidance is replaced arbitrarily with restorations. A functional adaptive guidance may become intolerable if suddenly changed.

If the anterior guidance is to be changed the requirements outlined in

Chapter 6 under Lateral Excursions and Protrusive Adjustment should be fulfilled, and can be summarised as follows:

Lateral excursions

Working side
(1) Canine guidance or group function, or canine guidance with the facility to drop into group function if change occurs.
(2) Smooth movement.
(3) Minimal deflection of the guide tooth/teeth.

Non-working side
Absence of contact.
Note that usually canine guidance cannot be built up to disclude the non-working side. The non-working side contacts must be reduced. Before reducing non-working side contacts, ensure that there are suitably positioned teeth on the working side, to pick up the guidance.

Protrusion
(1) Do not mutilate aesthetics.
(2) As many anterior teeth to contact as reasonable. Never just on upper lateral incisor.
(3) Smooth movement.
(4) Absence of posterior contact. (May not be possible in Class III occlusions.)

Small restorations such as Class III composite

In the absence of symptoms, it is rare for such restorations to alter the occlusion. The aim should be to copy the existing occlusal contacts. Any intercuspal contact should avoid the margin of the restoration. Preferably, protrusive contacts and latero-protrusive contacts should be on enamel and not restorative material so as to lessen the possibility of differential wear between the restoration and opposing tooth tissue (fig. 9.2).

Large restorations such as acid-etch Class IV composite

Similar to the Class III composite example, although it may be more difficult to provide excursive contacts on natural tooth. However, if posssible, ensure that occlusal contacts are not solely on the restoration, so

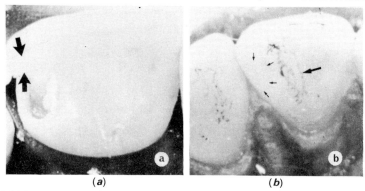

(a)   (b)

Fig. 9.2(a) Mesial cavity |1. Note the weakened incisal edge (*arrowed*). (b) Protrusive contacts on enamel 'skirt' around the restoration and avoid the weakened incisal edge.

as to reduce the chance of fracture and differential wear. In particular, in the edge-to-edge protrusive position, a single restoration should not bear the brunt of occlusal contact. Check that there is sufficient room for the composite in the ICP. If not, extend the preparation[1] (fig. 9.3).

Single anterior crown

Providing there is no previous adverse history, the restoration should harmonise with the existing occlusion. If there is a history of previous fracture, look at the posterior occlusion. Posterior deflective contacts causing an anterior slide of the mandible, resulting in contact between lower and upper incisors (particularly if on the fractured restoration) may indicate the need for occlusal adjustment prior to restoration, since it may be considered that the existing intercuspal position (at the end of the slide) leads to restorative material failure. As stated previously, if the slide from RCP to ICP has a large vertical and small horizontal component occlusal adjustment may be more readily undertaken since this is easy and predictable. Non-working side or posterior protrusive contacts associated with contact on the anterior tooth to be restored is an indication for localised posterior occlusal adjustment, prior to restoration, particularly if combined with muscle symptoms.

Pair of anterior crowns

In the absence of symptoms, the restorations should harmonise with the existing occlusion. With the history as above it may be decided to adjust the

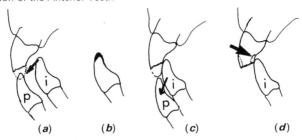

Fig. 9.3 Assessment for restoration of a fractured incisal edge. Saggital diagram through 1|
and 1| showing 1| in the ICP (i) and protrusive positions (p). (**a**) ICP.·The space between the
lingual of 1| and labial of 1| allows room for an acid-etch restoration. Protrusive position. 1|
passes through the projected incisal edge of 1|. Therefore 1| requires shortening as in (**b**).
(**c**) ICP. There is no space between the lingual of 1| and labial of 1|. Therefore modify the
preparation as in (**d**) (*arrow*). Protrusive position. 1| contacts projected incisal edge of 1|
therefore do not reduce 1|. (After Denehy *et al.*[1])

occlusion prior to restoration. However, with a grossly deranged occlusion
and an older patient who has adapted to this occlusion, it is prudent to
restore in harmony with the existing occlusion, rather than embark upon
extensive adjustment and/or restoration in order to alter an adaptive
functioning occlusion.

A simple technique for providing anterior crowns in harmony with the
existing occlusion (conformative) is to use the every-other-tooth technique.[2] In this technique one crown is prepared and an impression made
followed by the adjacent preparation and a second impression (fig. 9.4).
The technician then mounts the two upper working casts against the lower
cast, (figs 9.4(*b*) and (*c*) and using the one tooth preparation cast initially
(fig. 9.4(*d*)), obtains the mesio-distal and occlusal-cervical widths and
shape of lingual contour by copying the existing anterior guidance. The
crown can then be transferred to the two-tooth cast and the second crown
made using the first one as a guide (fig. 9.4(*e*)). In practice, the technician
may find it more convenient to go through all the stages for both crowns
simultaneously, thereby obtaining uniformity in the firing of the porcelain.
The type of jaw registration used in this technique is an intercuspal
registration taken at the correct vertical dimension (by definition). It may
be found unnecessary to use a recording medium if the casts can be hand
mounted.

Multiple anterior crowns

Shape of existing teeth acceptable
As for a pair of anterior crowns, it must be decided whether to adjust the

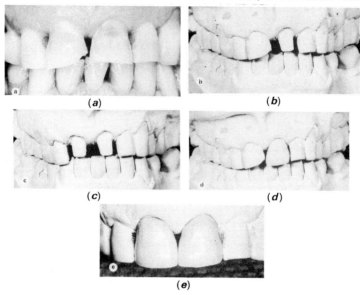

(a)   (b)

(c)   (d)

(e)

Fig. 9.4 Every other tooth technique for two anterior crowns. (a) 60-year-old patient requiring crowns of 1|1. (Conformative occlusion.) (b) One tooth preparation. Cast mounted. (c) Two teeth preparation. Cast mounted. (d) Crown on one tooth. Cast. (e) Finished crowns on two teeth cast.

posterior occlusion prior to restoration. If the anterior guidance is mainly on one anterior tooth, it may be advisable first to carry out small adjustments to this guidance so as to re-distribute it among several teeth. The use of the every-other-tooth technique simplifies the technical procedures and gives the technician much more information about tooth contour than he would have if all the anterior teeth were prepared and he was presented with a working cast of six anterior preparations.

Case history
The patient in figure 9.5 had undergone periodontal therapy and was happy with the shape of his heavily restored anterior teeth except for the long exposed roots. His upper partial denture required replacement and his lower arch needed restoring. In order to provide stability for the denture base it was decided to splint the upper anterior teeth which, following successful periodontal therapy and plaque control, were very mobile, due to reduced but healthy periodontium. Firstly 31|2 were prepared (fig. 9.5(a)), that is every other tooth, an impression taken and temporary crowns made. Then the remaining teeth were prepared and a second

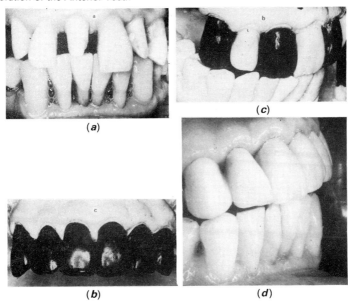

Fig. 9.5 Multiple anterior crowns, existing shape acceptable. (*a*) 31|2 prepared. (*b*) Every other tooth cast mounted and waxed. (*c*) Six wax patterns on multiple preparations cast. (*d*) Finished restorations.

impression taken of all six anterior teeth and temporaries made for them. Record bases were made on the working casts and at a subsequent visit jaw registrations were taken as follows: the temporaries were removed from 31|2 and a facebow registration made followed by a jaw registration taken in the intercuspal position with contact of the lower incisors against the upper temporary crowns. The first model was mounted on a Whipmix articulator with the facebow and then the lower cast mounted to the upper. The record base from the second preparation model was then placed in the mouth and a new intercuspal position jaw registration made, again using the temporary crowns to determine the correct vertical dimensions. The cast was then mounted to the already mounted lower. Every other tooth was then waxed to full contour on the first model (fig. 9.5(*b*)) and then transferred to the second model and the remaining teeth waxed (fig. 9.5(*c*)). The wax patterns were cut back to provide space for an even layer of porcelain and the castings were fabricated. Porcelain was then added using both casts. Figure 9.5(*d*) shows the final restorations.

Existing shape unacceptable

The shape may be unacceptable following advanced attrition, or gross tooth loss due to trauma or caries—it is frequently necessary to provide temporary restorations and adjust these prior to definitive restoration, the definitive restoration copying the temporaries. In order to make the correct diagnosis as to the shape of the temporary anterior crowns, it is necessary to have a stable posterior occlusion and absence of non-working side and posterior protrusive contacts (except Class III occlusions). This is achieved either through: acceptance of satisfactory existing posterior occlusion; occlusal adjustment; or temporary posterior restoration.

If the last opinion is required the temporaries must be well made preferably from cast metal so as to be durable. It should be understood that if posterior deflective contacts are present resulting in an anterior slide or displacement of the mandible it will be impossible to determine the form of the lingual surface of the anterior teeth with any certainty.

Although the criteria for anterior guidance on temporary crowns have not been investigated, it will be acceptable if the following are observed:

- A feeling of comfort as described by the patient.
- No increasing mobility of the teeth.
- No speech problems.
- Acceptable aesthetics.
- Stable temporary crowns (that is not becoming uncemented or broken).
- Smoothness of excursive movements as guided by the anteriors.

The temporary crowns may be adjusted by trimming with acrylic burs and/or direct build-up with auto-polymerising resin where necessary. Only when the above criteria are fulfilled are the temporaries copied, usually using the every other tooth technique.

Case presentation

The patient in figures 9.6 (*b*) and (*c*) drank two bottles of lemonade per day for three years, resulting in erosion almost into the pulp. Anterior temporary crowns were made initially from composite build-ups (fig. 9.6(*c*)) and then from prefabricated crown forms. The posterior occlusion had been previously stabilised by occlusal adjustment and temporary amalgam restorations (thereby also investigating the posterior teeth). The required shape of the lingual surface of the crown restorations was unknown. During a four-month period, the anterior temporary crowns were adjusted to fulfil the foregoing criteria. The anterior crowns were then copied as described for multiple anterior crowns. Subsequently, the posterior teeth were restored (figs. 9.6(*d*) and (*e*)).

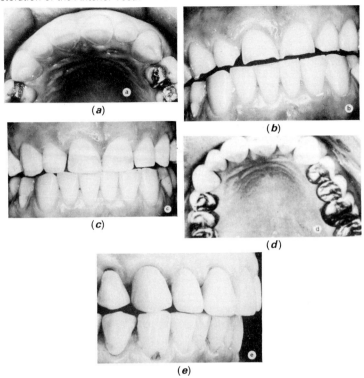

Fig. 9.6 Multiple crowns required but existing shape unacceptable. (*a*) Palatal view of 5|5. (*b*) Labial view. (*c*) Composite trial. (Note the posterior occlusion has been adjusted.) (*d*) Completed anterior and posterior restorations. (*e*) Completed restorations in right lateroprotrusive excursion.

An alternative method for reproducing the contours of the temporary crowns is as follows (fig. 9.7):

(1) Carefully clean the temporary crowns and position them on the working cast. If there is any binding on the die, bur out the inside of the crowns to ensure good seating, Observe the cast from the occlusal view and block out undercuts with soft wax.

(2) Paint plaster separating medium over the cast and crowns and then make a palatal plaster index of the crowns (impression plaster) keyed into the palatal half of the occlusal surfaces of the unprepared teeth. When set, check for ease of removal. Then reseat and paint separating medium over the index and make an additional index for the labial contours of the crowns. (Usually the labial index must be made in two halves, that is left and right to ensure removal. Alternatively use a silicone rubber index.)

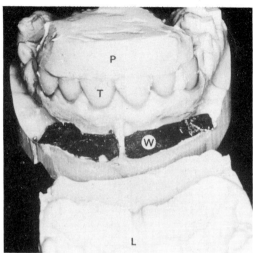

Fig. 9.7 Index used to copy anterior temporary crowns. Temporary crowns (T) on master cast. The palatal plaster index is in place, labial (L) removed. Wax block-out (W).

(3) Remove the temporary crowns from the cast and recement in the mouth. The technician can build wax into the indices to reproduce the shape. Note that it is imperative that the cast is mounted on an articulator in the intercuspal position, to obtain accurate contacts. Furthermore unless silver dies are used, it is safest to use separate master dies in case the working cast is damaged.

Multiple anterior restorations

Previous form is unknown and missing units present
As before, it is necessary to have a stable posterior occlusion first. Temporary anterior restorations are then fabricated either as a denture or temporary bridge.

Case report
The technique is best illustrated by the following case. The patient in figure 9.8(*a*) had lost the anterior teeth in a road traffic accident. Following occlusal adjustment a partial denture was provided (fig. 9.8(*b*)). Impressions were made of both the upper arch with its denture in place and the lower arch. These casts were mounted in the intercuspal position on a semi-adjustable articulator and the incisal pin lowered to touch the incisal table (fig. 9.8(*c*)). Cold-cure acrylic was flowed on to the table and as it began to set the casts were moved over each other using the teeth to guide

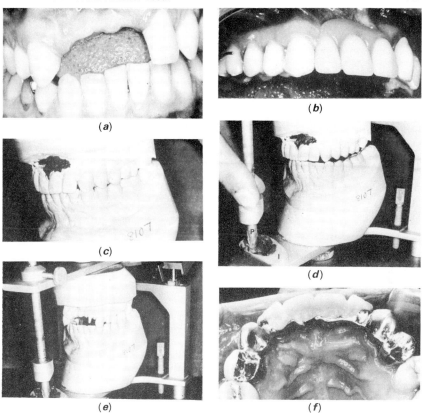

(a)

(b)

(c)

(d)

(e)

(f)

Fig. 9.8 Multiple anterior restorations. Previous form unknown and missing units present. (a) 21|1 lost following accident |2 subluxed. (b) Temporary denture and temporary crowns in place. (c) Cast of upper teeth and partial denture mounted against lower cast in the ICP (Posterior occlusion previously adjusted.) Whipmix articulator. (d) Incisal pin (P) moulding an acrylic anterior guidance table (I). (e) Upper working cast mounted to existing mounted lower cast (ICP). (f) Finished restorations.

the movement of the articulator. This resulted in the incisal pin moulding a guidance table in the polymerising acrylic (fig. 9.8(d)). This table was further refined with addition of more cold-cure acrylic so that the movement path of the pin in this plastic was dictated by the movement paths of the teeth on the study casts. The teeth were then prepared in the upper arch and working casts made and mounted again in the intercuspal position against the existing mounted lower working cast (fig. 9.8(e)). By using the incisal pin on the guidance table, the shape of the lingual concavity of the anterior teeth could be very closely approximated to that of the temporary

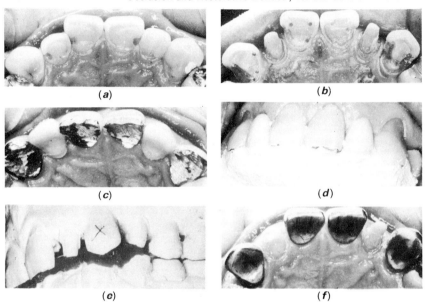

Fig. 9.9 Multiple anterior pinledges/threequarter crowns. (*a*) Palatal view of 321|123. (*b*) Preparation. (*c*) Temporary crowns in place. (*d*) Plaster index in mouth. Plaster added against temporary restorations. (*e*) Mounting casts with ICP registration. Note registration only between prepared/opposing teeth. (*f*) Final restorations tried in. Note the shape of the lingual concavity.

restoration so as to provide a similar anterior guidance (fig. 9.8(*f*)). The intercuspal mounting allowed for evenness of inter-arch contacts in the intercuspal position. If a temporary bridge had been used, reproduction would be facilitated by the index system described previously.

Multiple anterior pinledges and threequarter crowns

If the anterior lingual concavity is unknown, it will be necessary to reconstruct it with diagnostic restorations. Again, it is imperative to have a stable posterior occlusion. The clinical procedures are slightly different to the previous ones.

The patient, aged 58, had advanced attrition and erosion of the lingual surfaces of the upper anterior teeth, a history of bruxism, caries in anterior teeth and unsupported enamel at the incisal edges (fig. 9.9(*a*)). In the intercuspal position there was insufficient room for restorative material. Stage 1 was adjustment of the posterior occlusion to eliminate the anterior slide. This was followed by preparation of the anterior teeth (fig. 9.9(*b*)) and fabrication of cast gold temporary restorations made from direct

Duralay intra-oral patterns (fig. 9.9(c)). These castings were then cemented with temporary crown and bridge cement, and adjusted in the mouth so as to fulfil the criteria outlined where the existing shape is unacceptable. The lingual form was then copied as follows:

(1) Impression of the preparations.
(2) Fabrication of plaster index over working casts with space behind anterior teeth.
(3) Placement of temporary crowns in mouth.
(4) Plaster index inserted and plaster added to lingual surfaces of anterior temporaries (fig. 9.9(d)).
(5) Plaster and temporaries removed, and intercuspal jaw registration taken—by definition, at the correct vertical dimension (fig. 9.9(e)).
(6) Casts mounted. Plaster index placed on lingual of upper cast and wax flown in to give approximate contour of lingual surface of restorations.
(7) Intercuspal contacts established on mounted casts. Castings finished and sandblasted (fig. 9.9(f)).

The approach that has been outlined for the restoration of anterior teeth is a functional one, that is unless the existing form is accepted the new form of the lingual concavity is determined in the mouth.

Full mouth reconstruction

Sometimes the establishment of the lingual concavity can be facilitated by use of a fully adjustable articulator in which the condylar guidance is directly related to the form of the lingual concavity (fig. 9.10). Working casts are mounted in a programmed fully adjustable articulator and the form of the anterior teeth determined by aesthetic requirements and by moving the condylar elements. The crowns must be subsequently checked for functional acceptability during a period of temporary cementation.

Summary

The advantages of paying attention to the lingual form of the anterior teeth are as follows:
- Minimal adjustment required on the final restoration.
- Patient comfort and acceptability.
- Drifting of anterior teeth or increasing mobility due to occlusion may be prevented.
- Fractures of restorations due to the occlusion may be avoided.
- No subsequent uncontrolled change in anterior guidance influencing posterior occlusion.

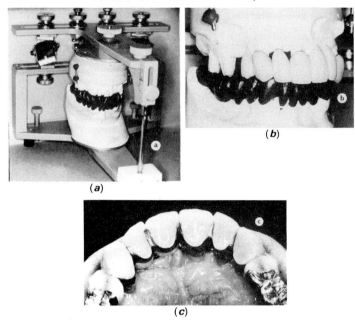

Fig. 9.10 Use of fully adjustable articulator to determined the anterior lingual concavity. (*a*) Waxing the restoration on the fully adjustable articulator. (*b*) Upper porcelain built to lower wax up. (Lowers subsequently built to completed uppers.) (*c*) Lingual shape of the anteriors has been determined by the condylar guidance and checked in the mouth.

In summary, decide whether to accept the existing posterior occlusion and anterior lingual concavity. If accepted, copy carefully. If altered ensure:

● Posterior stability.
● Absence of protrusive and latero-protrusive posterior contacts.
● Absence of non-working side contacts.
● Clinical acceptability of anterior guidance.
● That the anterior contacts are designed to minimise differential wear.
● That a decision is made re lateral guidance. Is it to be canine guidance or group function; or
● Canine guidance with the facility to 'drop into' group function if change occurs.

References

1 Denehy G E, Doering J V, Torney D L. Occlusion for successful Class IV acid etch restorations. *J Prosthet Dent* 1980; **44**: 274–278.
2 Dawson P E. *Evaluation, Diagnosis and Treatment of Occlusal Problems.* pp 177–180, St Louis: CV Mosby, 1974.

Duralay Inlay Resin: Cottrell & Co, Charlotte Street, London W1.

10 Questions and Answers

Because some questions probably remain unanswered, this book is concluded with some common questions and the author's answers.

Q *Can I stop a patient from grinding his teeth by adjusting the occlusion?*
A Although claims are made by clinicians that bruxism can be cured by occlusal treatment, there is sparse evidence to support this. It is ill-advised to suggest that a patient's bruxism will be cured: nevertheless, the location of specific teeth contacting during bruxism can be altered. Frequently the dentist can re-position contacts so as to direct occlusal loads through the teeth with the best support (to minimise mobility) and through the strongest parts of restorations and remaining tooth structure (to minimise mechanical failure), usually by occlusal adjustment and/or restorative and orthodontic therapy.

Q *Is wear due to bruxism or diet?*
A Studies have shown that tooth wear decreases with increasing urbanisation (see Bibliography). It is probable that much of the wear seen in the UK is not primarily diet related. Obviously if a dietary factor is suspected a detailed dietary history must be taken. If the teeth have an overall smooth glassy appearance plus attrition, check the diet for carbonated and citrus fruit drinks (fig. 10.1).

Q *How can a mobile tooth be considered healthy?*
A Studies (see Bibliography) have demonstrated that teeth with a reduced periodontium (remaining after the correction of advanced periodontitis)

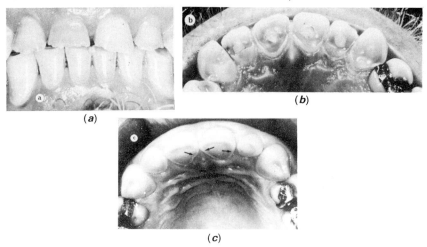

(b)

(a)

(c)

Fig. 10.1(*a*) and (*b*) Wear from bruxism. (*c*) Erosion showing smooth glassy approximal enamel ridge.

may be mobile although the periodontium is healthy. If a load is applied to a tooth, it will move until the 'normal slack' is taken up by the periodontium. In the absence of periodontitis, the support will extend almost to the amelocemental junction and hence the crown will not have moved very far by the time 'the slack' is taken up. However, following bone loss, if only the apical third of the tooth remains supported by periodontium, the crown would move further before the movement is limited even though in both cases the periodontium was of similar width.

Q *I was taught that the root surface of abutment teeth should equal or exceed that of the teeth replaced with pontics. Is this still valid?*
A Six-year follow-ups[1] have clearly demonstrated that the original teaching requires revision. Teeth with reduced but healthy periodontium can be used as abutments. However, this must be kept in perspective. The healthy periodontium (free from bleeding on probing, pink stippled gingivae, 0 to 3 mm crevice) is rarely seen in the UK.[2] This trend must be reversed so that teeth with healthy supporting tissues are used as bridge abutments. The use of minimal support in the presence of inflammation is courting failure. This does not imply that a large amount of support allows teeth with periodontitis to be used as bridge abutments since they will also fail. The answer therefore is to create first a healthy environment, and then decide upon abutment support.

Q *Should I reconstruct a patient's occlusion to treat TM pain?*
A No. Based on current knowledge it would be foolhardy. Firstly eliminate pain (if possible), preferably by reversible methods, such as occlusal splints or muscle exercises. If the patient requires occlusal reconstruction for other reasons (such as missing teeth, fractures, lost restorations) then only do this when the patient has been symptom-free for a reasonable period of time (for example 9 months).

Q *My patient has loose teeth and wants them splinted. Should I not crown and splint them immediately?*
A The first question is: why are they loose? Nothing is gained by immediate splinting other than a feeling of firmness of teeth. Obviously in advanced periodontitis this may be necessary. However, usually such an approach is unnecessary since resolution of inflammation will reduce mobility which should then be reassesed (it may no longer concern the patient), occlusal adjustment may reduce the mobility to acceptable levels and splinting may commit the patient to unnecessary expensive dentistry. Unless carefully carried out, splinting will result in unnecessary problems.

Remember to eliminate periodontitis first and then reassess mobility. Mobility is a symptom or sign, not a disease.

Q *How long should an occlusal splint be worn?*
A The splint should be worn for as much of the day and night as possible. Probably to start with it should be removed at mealtimes. Obviously it should be removed for social occasions, when it would be embarrassing. It should be worn and adjusted until symptoms subside. The patient can then re-use it as and when necessary unless its use was primarily to relax the musculature prior to diagnostic mounting of study casts or prior to restoration. In the former case it is discarded, while in the latter it is worn until occlusal adjustment is commenced.

Q *I always have difficulty in guiding the mandible to the retruded contact position on my patients. What should I do?*
A Much of the difficulty is due to inexperience and lack of confidence. It is essential to make the patient feel calm, relaxed and secure. If you 'bang the mandible about on a deflective contact', the patient will immediately tighten up. If possible, cradle the patient's head between your arms and chest to give this feeling of security and to prevent the head from shaking around. Practise on colleagues, staff or friends before starting on patients.

The other reason for the difficulty is that the patient has adapted to his occlusion, but the musculature is now 'programmed' to avoid deflective contacts. He will not allow the mandible to be manipulated to the RCP. Such patients require some form of conditioning, for example by an anterior jig or occlusal splint, before the mandible can be easily manipulated. Although the mandibular–maxillary relationship is termed retruded, remember that current practice is to manipulate the mandible so that the condyles are in their most superior relationships to the fossae.

Q *Is the RCP stable?*
A The RCP varies from one time of day to another, and from one technique to another (see Bibliography). For a particular operator using a single technique, it is sufficiently reproducible over the treatment period to make it a useful clinical reference point. If an occlusion is to be reorganised, it enables the dentist and technician to provide even, simultaneous contact of all posterior teeth. As stated by Celenza in 1978, 'replicability is a strong requirement for clinical management of the refinement of the occlusion. The relative replicability of the condylar position allows for a confirmation of the registration. This is important only in that it facilitates precision at the occlusal level. All indications point to a small acceptable range of condylar positioning at the posterior superior slope of the eminentia.'

Q *How do I start applying the principles of occlusion in my practice?*
A Start preferably by practising on colleagues. Improve your examination procedures. As you see more you will understand and question more. Start occlusal adjustments on teeth that you will be restoring anyway, so that nothing is lost in the learning. For example, if 6| requires a crown, mark the occlusal contacts, reshape the areas, and mark again. Note what happens and then prepare the crown. Preferably mount study casts on an articulator and carry out mock adjustment. Acknowledge that learning takes time.

Q *What occlusion should I aim for on amalgams?*
A The occlusion will be conformative or reorganised.
   If *conformative*, it fits in with the existing jaw relationships. If possible do a minimal amalgam so as to cause minimal disruption of the occlusion. When this is not possible, aim for contact in the intercuspal position (ICP), preferably located over the centre of the tooth, with absence of protrusive, non-working and retruded contacts. Decide whether to provide working contacts on the amalgam—usually these are undesirable since they will result in fracture.

If *reorganised,* the occlusion will have been adjusted to eliminate the slide from RCP to ICP. If, on completion of adjustment, RCP and ICP are different, aim for contact in RCP as well as ICP, ensuring that this does not reintroduce a slide from RCP to ICP.

Q *What do I actually do when carving an amalgam?*
A First decide whether the approach is conformative or reorganised. Always adjust an over-erupted opposing cusp. Choose an amalgam with a high initial compressive strength (for example, spherical or dispersal phase alloys). After packing wait at least 3 minutes. Carve the amalgam, but leave it slightly undercarved (that is, high). Ask the patient to close gently until the teeth 'meet the most'. High spots will be shiny. Carve upper amalgams from 1 mm distal to the mark up to and including it, to allow the mandible to move to the RCP. Carve lower amalgams from 1 mm mesial to the mark up to and including it, for the same reason. It may be necessary to mark with tapes. Once the ICP is established, check lateral and protrusive excursions: eliminate all but the ICP contacts. Check RCP to ICP and eliminate contact if necessary (see the previous question and answer).

Q *I recently prepared* $\overline{7654|}$ *for full coverage (* $\overline{8|}$ *missing). After making the impression I asked the patient to close and found* $7|\overline{7|}$ *in contact. Why?*
A The intercuspal position was probably anterior to the RCP. The condyle was not fully seated in the fossa. Preparation of the quadrant eliminated all of the deflective contacts and allowed the condyles to move superiorly under muscle load, thereby eliminating the space created by tooth preparation. The deflective contacts should have been removed on the right quadrant several weeks before tooth preparation (fig. 10.2).

Q *My temporary bridge* $\overline{7-5|}$ *was continually uncementing. When the final bridge returned from the laboratory it was high on* $7|\overline{7|}$. *I know the teeth have not moved, since the bridge fitted. What did the technician do wrong?*
A The technician probably did nothing wrong. Assuming that the temporaries were well made and the preparations reasonable, the lack of cementation implies that:

(1) They did not reproduce exactly the original occlusal contacts (almost impossible), or

(2) The mandibular–maxillary relationships were altering, that is adapting to the altered occlusion, or

(3) By the time the bridge was fitted, the condyle was positioned more superiorly in the fossa, thus reducing space between the preparations and

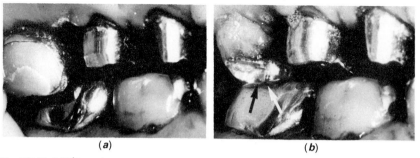

(a)   (b)

Fig. 10.2(a) 65| have been prepared. (**b**) On removing the existing crown on 7| and asking the patient to close, the 7| preparation and 7| crown were found to be in contact.

the opposing teeth. Adjustment should have been made as above or on the temporary until a stable state had been reached prior to jaw registration.

Q *Why do anterior teeth drift in middle-aged patients?*
A This is poorly investigated. Clincally it appears to be due to an alteration in the balance between musculature on the labial, forces from the lingual (tongue and occlusal) and tooth support (crown:root ratio). The aetiology may be multifactorial, but is commonly due to (1) periodontitis (reduced support leads to increased crown:root ratios), (2) posterior deflective contacts leading to an anterior path of closure and increased loading of 3|3, (3) loss of posterior occlusal support, (4) reduced elasticity of circumoral tissues with ageing, (5) altered crown contours (labial and palatal) particularly on bonded porcelain restorations, or (6) a habit such as pencil biting.

Q *Why do some patients tolerate high fillings whereas others constantly complain about minute spots?*
A Two factors appear to influence the response: occlusal contacts and central nervous system response. The threshold for tolerance varies between people and within the same person at different times. For example, stress can affect the level such that a patient who previously accepted an adaptive occlusion suddenly becomes aware of small changes associated with new restorations.

Q *Why does occlusal adjustment in a patient with a large horizontal but small vertical dimension between RCP and ICP sometimes result in squeaking sounds?*
A The end result of the large horizontal/small vertical dimension is

frequently absence of anterior guidance. The large rubbing areas often present on the posterior teeth contact in lateral excursions and squeak.

Q *Can and should anterior guidance always be provided?*
A Anterior guidance, although desirable, cannot always be provided. In such cases try and provide for the guidance to be as far forward of the posterior teeth as possible.

Q *What sort of articulator should I buy to start with?*
A A semi-adjustable one with a simple facebow system. The Whipmix, Dentatus, Denar Mark II articulators should perhaps be considered.

Q *My technician always seems to mount the casts wrongly. What should I do?*
A Mount them yourself until you are certain that it is not your registration that is wrong. Are you taking a tooth-apart registration and not using a facebow? If so, closure through the thickness of the registration may be introducing errors. Perhaps you are capturing a position distal to the ICP in which case only a few teeth will contact making a correct mounting appear incorrect.

Q *What are the most important points to remember when mounting casts for diagnosis?*
A Use the retruded position, but do not allow any tooth contact. Check the accuracy of the registration, that is no distortion; use a facebow.

Q *What are the most important points to remember when mounting casts for restoration?*
A Whenever possible use the intercuspal position, that is teeth together maximally meshed. However, do not ask the patient to squeeze tightly lest the unprepared teeth are displaced relative to the prepared tooth (which is out of occlusion). Check the accuracy of the registration on the casts.

Q *You say that wax is a poor material to use if any delay is anticipated between making a registration and mounting the casts (Chapter 5). What should I use?*
A Wherever possible, casts should be mounted at the chairside. If a delay is anticipated, then use zinc oxide and eugenol bite registration paste carried on a soft metal carrier, or use Duralay. It is the dentist's responsibility to check the mounting, so time should be programmed for this procedure.

Q *I have heard that zinc stearate may be poisonous. Is this true?*
A No. According to the *Condensed Chemical Dictionary*[4] zinc stearate is non-toxic. It appears that zinc stearate may be damaging to infants if inhaled,[5] but there is no reference to adults.

Q *How important is immediate side shift?*
A There are no studies available which clarify this point. Clinically, it is a complicating factor particularly when cast or porcelain posterior restorations are required for a patient with a shallow anterior guidance and short posterior teeth. Diagnostic instruments are now becoming available which enable the clinician to determine whether immediate sideshift is present without requiring a full pantographic survey.[3]

Q *What influence does the curve of Spee have?*
A A patient with a steep curve of Spee will have less room between the posterior teeth in protrusive and lateral excursive movements than a patient with a shallow curve. Therefore shallow anterior guidance, shallow condylar guidance, immediate sideshift, plus steep curve of Spee leaves little room for cusps.

Q *Are cusps necessary?*
A The masticatory efficiency of cusped rather than cuspless fixed restorations has not been investigated. I consider that cusps and fossae are important in certain types of restorations from the standpoint of stability and wear, although again, neither has been investigated. Many studies have reported that tooth wear is natural in primitive man. However, he did not have teeth restored with modern restorative materials—none of which wears at the same rate as teeth—so it is difficult to extrapolate the findings to modern man, who requires tooth restoration and who finds excessively worn anterior teeth socially unacceptable.

Single unsplinted units require more stabilisation from the occlusion than do splinted units. Both types require 'non-rubbing' types of occlusion if wear is to be minimised (not researched) and mechanical failures minimised (not researched). Cusps fitting into shallow fossae provide the stabilising contacts and allow for non-rubbing lateral movements through escape grooves. It is the practitioner's responsibility to prescribe the form of occlusal surfaces required for each specific restoration.

Q *Should all patients have their occlusions adjusted?*
A There must be a definite reason for adjusting an occlusion. Essentially there are two indications:

(1) Relief of symptoms and signs, for example drifting anterior teeth or increasing mobility.

(2) Convenience. If multiple posterior restorations are required for a patient with a large vertical/small horizontal slide it is easier to adjust before restoration than on each restoration. However, a large horizontal/ small vertical slide may be better left alone. Use common sense and practise on mounted casts.

Q *When is an occlusal adjustment/equilibration complete?*
A An occlusal equilibration is never complete since a check must be made at each recall and any necessary small adjustments made. An adjustment prior to restoration is complete when the patient is comfortable over several months, the mandible is easily manipulated and there is even contact over the majority of teeth in the RCP. Tooth preparation can then be carried out.

Q *What should I use for temporaries?*
A Any material that fits well, has good contour, is stable for the period required, maintains the occlusal contacts, maintains approximal contacts, can be cemented and readily removed, is not irritant, and is aesthetic when required. Acrylic temporaries fulfil most of these requirements except if prolonged use is required or if free monomer is present which would be an irritant.

For posterior teeth I use a range of temporaries depending upon circumstances:

(1) Single to 3 units. A matrix is made from a study cast or casts of diagnostic waxing (fig. 10.3) and temporaries made directly with one of the temporary crown and bridge resins.

(2) Four or more units. Shell crowns are used. Alginate impressions are made of diagnostic casts or waxing; reinforcing wires are placed in the occlusal surface and acrylic poured (fig. 10.4) and cured in a pressure pot. The solid block of temporaries is removed and polished and the insides drilled out with a tungsten carbide bur. They are relined in the mouth. Note that diagnostic waxing must be thick in the cervical region to give bulk to the temporary crowns.[6]

(3) Multiple units for long term temporaries (provisional restorations 2 months to 18 months). Use metal castings (for example gold or semi or non-precious metal) and acrylic and metal. Take two impressions, pour one in Divestment and one in stone; wax copings on Divestment model and cast (fig. 10.5). Transfer to mounted casts and wax, and process acrylic on to

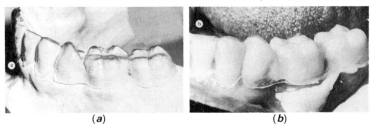

(a)   (b)

Fig. 10.3(a) Matrix from study cast or diagnostic wax for single to three units. (b) Filled with crown and bridge resin and temporary made directly in mouth.

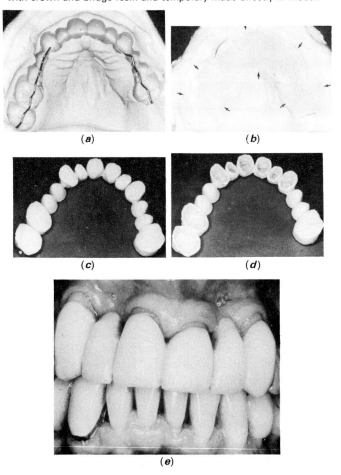

(a)   (b)

(c)   (d)

(e)

Fig. 10.4 Fabrication of a shell bridge. (a) Reinforcing wire positioned in alginate impression of a diagnostic cast. (b) Acrylic poured in. (c) Solid block removed. (d) Potential preparations drilled out. (e) Relined in mouth. (Note 2|2 extracted.)

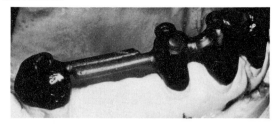

Fig. 10.5 Waxing copings on Divestment model. (Divestment is a refractory investment.)

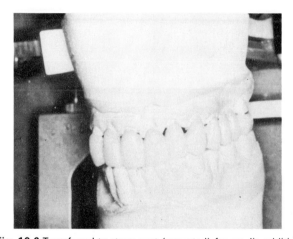

Fig. 10.6 Transferred to stone cast (mounted) for acrylic addition.

casting (fig. 10.6). Units not requiring acrylic can be made in Duralay, checked in the mouth for contacts (fig. 10.7) and cast and cemented. Metal can be reclaimed when the definitive restorations are provided.

Q *My technician uses removable dies. Sometimes these exhibit play. How can the occlusion be right and what should I do?*
A I prefer to use a two-impression technique without removable dies (easiest with reversible hydrocolloids). Take a quadrant impression and make individual dies (fig. 10.8). The pins are purely for storage in the wooden block. Take a full arch impression, then pour and mount the solid casts (fig. 10.8). Wax the initial copings on the individual dies, transfer to master cast, complete waxing up of contour and occlusion, replace on individual dies, finish margins, invest and cast.

With some rubber impression materials use two pours from a single impression to make individual dies and master casts.

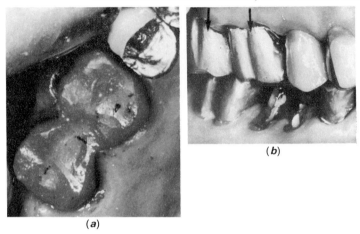

(b)

(a)

Fig. 10.7(a) Checking Duralay temporaries in the mouth for contacts. (**b**) Duralay has been invested and cast and now cemented in mouth.

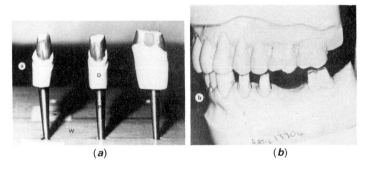

(a)   (b)

Fig. 10.8(a) Individual dies. (D=die, P=pin, W=wooden block.) (**b**) Full arch cast.

Q *What is a remount procedure for fixed restorations?*
A The castings are tried in the mouth, and new retruded registrations made usually with an anterior jig in place (fig. 10.9(a)). A pick-up impression is made and new casts fabricated containing the casting. These are remounted in the articulator (fig. 10.9(b)) and the occlusion refined. Frequently the remount is performed after several months of temporary cementation of the castings.

Q *What are the alternatives for patients with advanced attrition?*
A This depends upon the clinical state (for example, number and location of teeth or periodontal condition); the age and medical condition of the

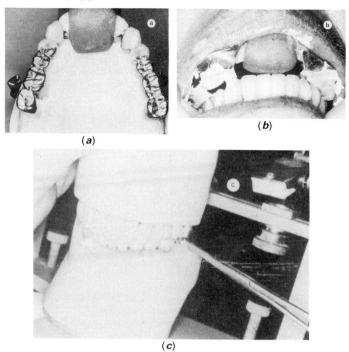

(a)

(b)

(c)

Fig. 10.9 Part of remount procedure. (*a*) Anterior jig made on final castings. (*b*) Transferred to the mouth and new jaw registrations made. (*c*) New casts made and remounted with the jaw registration. The occlusion is refined.

patient; the desires of the patient; the clinical ability and technical back-up; finance. The possible approaches are: (1) Simple patch-up and repairs as necessary. Breakdown will continue so ensure that both you and the patient are aware of this. (2) Overlay dentures (fig. 10.10). (3) Posterior overlay dentures plus anterior crowns. These are dangerous if anteriors are restored with post crowns, since if a posterior denture is not worn the anterior roots may split. (4) Full mouth reconstruction.

Q *Is it justifiable to adjust an opposing tooth when cementing a restoration?*
A Yes, provided it is planned and not an afterthought! For example, if for some reason an over-erupted opposing cusp is not shortened at preparation, shorten it on the opposing cast. Do the same in the mouth. If the fossa of the restoration were to be deepened on cementation, the over-erupted opposing cusp would form a non-working side contact against the restoration.

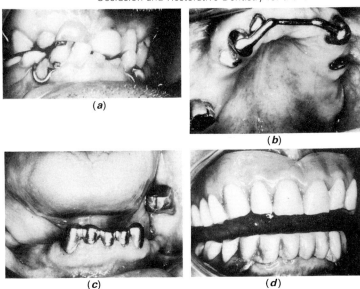

Fig. 10.10(a) The patient had advanced attrition and a severe retching problem. (**b**) Upper arch. Copings and bars for retention of upper overlay denture. 4|5 had been previously root treated, and they were cut flush with the gingivae and occluded with amalgam. (Each had two thin roots which precluded post placement.) (**c**) Copings in lower arch. (**d**) Overlay dentures 1 year after fitting. The 3|3 are reinforced internally with castings that fit over the copings. The upper is a horseshoe design.

Q *Will not treatment take a long time if I think about mobility, periodontitis, and occlusion?*
A Yes, it will, but what is the hurry? The aim should be to move progressively towards a maintainable state of health. Obviously acute lesions should be treated, but thereafter many restorative plans of treatment can be spread over a long period, only moving from one stage to the next as the objectives of each stage are achieved. Frequently the treatment is modified at each reassessment stage, and progression to the next stage is no longer required.

Q *Could you please give me a guide to full mouth restoration?*
A Stabilise the posterior occlusion. Determine the anterior guidance on provisional restoration. Copy the anterior guidance on definitive anterior restorations. Restore the posterior teeth.

Q *In a nutshell, what are some of the concepts of full mouth rehabilitation?*
A All concepts require a healthy periodontium: we consider five of them.

(1) *Gnathological concept*   The movements of the condyles in the fossae determine occlusal form. There should be simultaneous contact of all posterior teeth in RCP with forces directed through the long axes. RCP and ICP should be coincident. In any excursive or protrusive movement, the anterior or canine guidance should separate (disclude) the posteriors. If anterior guidance cannot be provided, place it as far forward as possible. The lingual concavity of the anterior teeth is determined by condylar guidance. The case must be waxed on a fully adjustable articulator. (This approach is particularly useful for wear cases with individual units, and a large vertical/small horizontal discrepancy between RCP and ICP.) Cusp fossa–tripod contacts are provided.

(2) *Freedom in centric concept*   As Ramfjord has written:[7] 'this advocates a small flat area on a horizontal plane between the retruded contact position and intercuspal position ("long centric") and with occlusal functional guidance leading to the intercuspal position rather than to the retruded position. The distance between the retruded contact position and the intercuspal position in this system is not critical, but usually approximately 0·5 mm ± 0·3 mm.' According to Dawson,[8] the area of freedom is allowed on the anterior teeth without provision of the horizontal table on the posteriors.

(3) *Pankey–Mann–Schuyler concept*   The anterior guidance is determined functionally. The anteriors and lower posteriors are restored (fig. 10.11). A functionally generated path (FGP) technique is used to assist waxing of the upper posterior restorations. The aim is to have simultaneous contact of all posterior teeth, absence of non-working side contact, group function on the working side (although some operators aim for canine disclusion) with an area of freedom to be provided anterior to RCP (not more than 0·5 mm). A simple measuring system is used to determine the

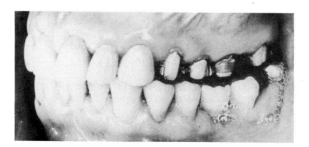

Fig. 10.11 The upper anteriors and lower posteriors have been restored. The upper posterior quadrants are prepared. An FGP can now be made and the upper wax patterns completed.

occlusal plane. A fully adjustable articulator is not required. It can be used for individual units and is particularly useful for splinted units when there is no increased mobility. Movement of teeth while making an FGP registration compromises the registration.

(4) *Yuodelis concept* for advanced periodontitis cases (fig. 10.12). The foundation of a healthy periodontium is stressed. The aim is for simultaneous contacts of posterior teeth in RCP (usually coincident with ICP) with forces through the long axes of teeth. Anterior disclusion for protrusive and canine disclusion for lateral excursion. Lateral contacts are arranged such that if the canine disclusion is lost through wear or tooth movement the posterior teeth drop into group function. Much information is gained from diagnostic temporary restorations.

Sometimes one arch of preparations is mounted against the cast of the

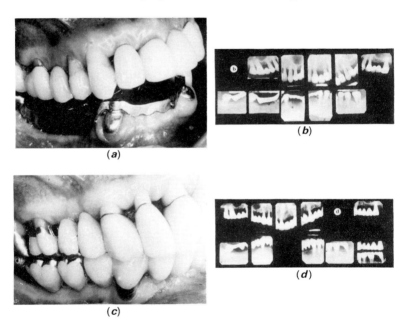

(a)

(b)

(c)

(d)

Fig. 10.12 (a) and (b) Advanced periodontitis has resulted in Grade III mobility and inability to function satisfactorily with existing prostheses. Treatment was aimed initially at removing plaque-induced inflammation, correcting pockets and re-establishing jaw relationships, subsequently followed by reconstruction. (c) and (d) For this patient RCP and ICP were coincident. Canine guidance was provided for lateral excursions and cusp fossa contacts provided in the ICP. The units were splinted because the unsplinted mobility remaining, following the correction of the periodontitis, was unacceptable to the patient. (Periodontal surgery by Mr J. Zamet and endodontics by Mr E Nicholls.)

opposing temporary restorations (made from a diagnostic waxing). On completion the opposing arch is restored to this already restored arch. Both fully and semi-adjustable articulators are used: 'use the right instrument for the case in hand'. Emphasis is placed on margin placement and crown contour.

(5) *Nyman and Lindhe concept* for extremely advanced periodontitis cases. The foundation is a healthy though reduced periodontium. Provide an even contact in ICP although no great emphasis is placed upon the type of contacts. When distal support is present use anterior guidance for protrusive and canine disclusion for lateral excursions. When long tooth-borne cantilevered restorations are provided arrange for balanced occlusion, that is simultaneous working and non-working side contacts on the cantilever. All restorations should be fabricated on semi-adjustable articulators with average settings and emphasis on supragingival margin placement. Monthly recall appointments with a hygienist are required for maintenance.

Q *When adjusting a non-working side contact, I am unsure of what to look for on the working side.*
A Although there are many situations in which non-working side contacts should be removed, remember that contact must be established on the working side so that working side teeth provide the guidance and the non-working side contacts can be 'cleared out'. Sometimes there are no suitably positioned teeth on the working side, and unless this were checked before adjustment to the non-working side, you might find that you were grinding more and more off the non-working side, never being able to eliminate the contact.

Q *Is resistance to periodontitis always associated with thick tissue, as implied in Chapter 2?*
A No. The relationship of tissue thickness to progression of periodontitis has not been well studied. However, a common clinical impression is that patients who have advanced attrition tend to have the clinical appearance of thick firm gingivae with the teeth set into thick bone.

Q *I cannot possibly apply the things you have said. I have no time and my patients will not accept it.*
A It is the responsibility of the profession to keep up to date. Obviously compromises are required by individual circumstances, but compromise should emanate from knowledge, not from ignorance.

References

1 Nyman S, Lindhe J, Lundgren D. The role of occlusion for the stability of fixed bridges in patients with reduced periodontal tissue support. *J Clin Periodontol* 1975; **2**: 53–66.
2 Sheiham A. The epidemiology of dental caries and periodontal disease. *J. Clin Periodontol* 1979; **6**: 7–15.
3 Lundeen H. Mandibular movement recordings and articulator adjustments simplified. *Dent Clin North Am* 1979; **23**: 231–241.
4 Hawkey. *Condensed chemical dictionary.* 10th ed. London: Van Nostrand, Reinhold, 1981.
5 Abt T. Inhalation of zinc stearate. *J Am Med Assoc* 1925; **84**: 750–754.
6 Schluger S, Yuodelis R A, Page R C. *Periodontol disease.* p 643. Philadelphia: Lea and Febiger, 1977.
7 Ramfjord S P. Is it really necessary to record jaw movements? *Quintessence Int* 1982; **13**: 187–193.
8 Dawson P E. In *Occlusion, the state of the art.* Celenza F V, Nasedkin J N (ed). p 42. Chicago: Quintessence, 1978.

Divestment: Whip-Mix Corporation, 361 Farmington Avenue, Louisville, Kentucky 40217, USA.
Duralay: Reliance Dental Manufacturing Co, Worth, Illinois 60482, USA.

Bibliography

Further general reading

Arnold N R, Frumker S C. *Occlusal treatment.* Philadelphia: Lea and Febiger, 1976.

Dawson P E. *Evaluation, diagnosis and treatment of occlusal problems.* St Louis: C V Mosby, 1974.

Ramfjord S P, Ash M M. *Occlusion.* 2nd ed. Philadelphia: W B Saunders, 1971.

Schluger S, Yuodelis R A, Page R C. *Periodontal disease: basic phenomena, clinical management and occlusal and restorative interrelationships.* Philadelphia: Lea and Febiger, 1977.

Shillinburg H T, Hobo S, Whitsett L D. *Fundamentals of fixed prosthodontics.* Chicago: Quintessence, 1978.

Zarb G A, Carlsson G E. *Temporomandibular joint function and dysfunction.* Copenhagen: Munksgaard, 1979.

Classified bibliography

Anatomy and physiology

Posselt U. *Physiology of occlusion and rehabilitation.* 2nd ed. Oxford: Blackwell, 1968.

Ramfjord S P, Ash M M. *Occlusion.* 2nd ed, pp 4–109. Philadelphia: W. B. Saunders, 1971.

Tooth wear

Baer M J. Dimensional changes in the human head and face in the third decade of life. *Am J Phys Anthropol* 1956; **14**: 557–575.

Berry D C, Poole D F G. Masticatory function and oral rehabilitation. *J Oral Rehabil* 1974; **1**: 191–205.

Berry D C, Poole D F G. Attrition: possible mechanisms of compensation. *J Oral Rehabil* 1976; **3**: 201–206.

Beyron H L. Occlusal changes in adult dentition. *J Am Dent Assoc* 1954; **48**: 674–686.

Davies T G H, Pedersen P O. The degree of attrition of the deciduous teeth and first permanent molars of primitive and urbanised Greenland natives. *Br Dent J* 1955; **99**: 35–43.

Goose D H. Dental measurement: an assessment of its value in anthropological studies. In *Dental anthropology*. Brothwell D R (ed). pp 125–148. Oxford: Pergamon Press, 1963.

McNammara J A. Independent functions of the two heads of the lateral pterygoid muscle. *Am J Anat* 1973; **138**: 197–205.

Molnar S. Human tooth wear, tooth function and cultural variability. *Am J Phys Anthropol* 1971; **34**: 175–189.

Murphy T. Compensatory mechanisms in facial height adjustment to functional tooth attrition. *Aust Dent J* 1959; **4**: 312–323.

Sicher H. The biology of attrition. *Oral Surg* 1953; **6**: 406–412.

Williamson E H, Woelfel J B, Williams B H. A longitudinal study of rest position and centric occlusion. *Angle Orthod* 1975; **45**: 130–136.

Adaptive changes (see also Tooth Wear)

Butler J H, Stallard R E. Effect of occlusal relationships on neurophysiological pathways. *J Periodont Res* 1969; **4**: 141–151.

Butler J H, Stallard R E. Physiologic stress and tooth contact. *J Periodont Res* 1969; **4**: 152–158.

Celenza F V. Position Paper. In *Occclusion: the state of the art*. Celenza F V, Nasedkin J N (ed). pp 31–41. Chicago: Quintessence, 1978.

Durkin J F, Heely J D, Irving J T. Cartilage of the mandibular condyle. In *Temporomandibular joint function and dysfunction*. Zarb G A, Carlsson G E (ed). pp 43–100. Copenhagen: Munksgaard, 1979.

Moffett B C, Johnson L C, McCabe J D Asqew H C. Articular remodelling in the adult human TMJ. *Am J Anat* 1964; **115**: 119–142.

Ramfjord S P, Ash M M. *Occlusion*. 2nd ed, pp 44–109. Philadelphia: W B Saunders, 1971.

Schaerer P, Stallard R E, Zander H A. Occlusal interferences and mastication: an electro-myographic study. *J Prosthet Dent* 1967; **17**: 438–449.

Vollmer W H, Rateitschack K H. Influence of occlusal adjustment by grinding on gingivitis and mobility of traumatised teeth. *J Clin Periodontol* 1975; **2**: 113–124.

Weinberg L A. Radiographic investigations into temporomandibular joint function. *J Prosthet Dent* 1975; **33**: 672–688.

Bruxism

Greene C S, Lerman M D, Sutcher H D, Laskin D M. The TMJ pain dysfunction syndrome: heterogeneity of the patient population. *J Am Dent Assoc* 1969; **79**: 1168–72.

Nadler S P. The importance of bruxing. *J Oral Med* 1968; **23**: 142–148.

Ramfjord S P. Bruxism: a clinical and electromyographic study. *J Am Dent Assoc* 1961; **62**:21–44.

Ramfjord S P, Ash M M. *Occlusion*. 2nd ed, pp 113–124. Philadelphia: W. B. Saunders, 1971.

Rugh J D, Solberg W K. Psychological implications in temporomandibular pain and dysfunction. In *Temporomandibular joint function and dysfunction*. Zarb G A, Carlsson G E (ed). pp 252–264. Copenhagen: Munksgaard, 1979.

Yemm R. Neurophysiologic studies of temporomandibular joint dysfunction. In *Temporomandibular joint function and dysfunction*. (ed). Zarb G A Carlsson G E, pp 230–234. Copenhagen: Munksgaard, 1979.

Mobility/Periodontitis

Glickman I, Smulow J B. The combined effects of inflammation and trauma from occlusion in periodontitis. *Int Dent J* 1969; **19**: 393–407.

Lindhe J, Svanberg G. Influence of trauma from occlusion on progression of experimental periodontitis in the Beagle dog. *J Clin Periodontol* 1974; **1**: 3–14.

Nyman S, Lindhe J, Lundgren D. The role of occlusion for the stability of fixed bridges in patients with reduced periodontal tissue support. *J Clin Periodontol* 1975; **2**: 53–66.

Nyman S, Lindhe J, Ericson I. The effect of progressive tooth mobility on destructive periodontitis. *J Clin Periodontol* 1978; **5**: 213–225.

O'Leary T J. Tooth mobility. *Dent Clin North Am* 1969; **13**: 567–579.

Polson A M. Inter-relationship of inflammation and tooth mobility (trauma), *in* Pathogenesis of periodontal disease. *J Clin Periodontol* 1980; **7**: 351–360.

Polson A M, Zander H A. Occlusal traumatism. In *Advances in occlusion*. Edit Lundeen H, Gibbs C. Bristol: Wright, 1982.

Stoller N H, Laudenbach K W. Clinical standardisation of horizontal tooth mobility. *J Clin Periodontol* 1980; 7: 242–250.

Vollmer W H, Rateitschack K H. Influence of occlusal adjustment by grinding on gingivitis and mobility of traumatised teeth. *J Clin Periodontol* 1975; 2: 113–125.

Waerhaug J. The angular bone effect and its relationship to trauma from occlusion and downgrowth of subgingival plaque. *J Clin Periodontol* 1979; 6: 61–82.

Variability of retruded contact position

Celenza F V. Centric position: replacement and character. *J Prosthet Dent* 1973; 30: 591–598.

Grasso J E, Sharry J. The duplicability of arrowpoint tracings in dentulous subjects. *J Prosthet Dent* 1968; 20: 106–115.

Helkimo M, Ingervall B, Carlsson G E. Variation of retruded and muscular position of mandible under different recording conditions. *Acta Odontol Scand* 1971; 29: 423–437.

Hoffman P J, Silverman S I, Garfinkel L. Comparison of condylar position in centric relation and in centric occlusion in dentulous subjects. *J Prosthet Dent* 1973; 30: 582–588.

Kantor M E, Silverman S I, Garfinkel L. Centric relation recording techniques: a comparative investigation. *J. Prosthet Dent* 1972; 28: 593–600.

Long J H. Location of the terminal hinge axis by intra-oral means. *J. Prosthet Dent* 1970; 23: 11–24.

Lundeen H C. Centric relation records: the effect of muscle action. *J. Prosthet Dent* 1974; 31: 244–251.

Noble W H. Antero-posterior position of myomonitor centric. *J. Prosthet Dent* 1975; 33: 398–403.

Omar R, Wise M D. Mandibular flexure associated with muscle force applied in the retruded axis position. *J Oral Rehabil* 1981; 8: 209–221.

Posselt U. Studies in the mobility of the human mandible. *Acta Odontol Scand* 1952; 10: Suppl 10.

Shafagh I, Yoder J L, Thayer K E. Diurnal variance of centric relation position. *J. Prosthet Dent* 1975; 34: 574–582.

Strohaver R A. A comparison of articulator mountings made with centric relation and myocentric position records. *J. Prosthet Dent* 1972; 28: 378–390.

Teo C S, Wise M D. Comparison of retruded axis articulator mountings with and without applied muscular force. *J Oral Rehabil* 1981; 8: 363–376.

Lateral excursions

Beyron H. Optimal occlusion. *Dent Clin North Am* 1969; **13**: 537–554.

Granger E R. *Practical procedures in oral rehabilitation.* Philadelphia: Lipincott, 1962.

Lauritzen A G. *Atlas of occlusal analysis.* Colorado Springs: HAH Publications, 1974.

Schluger S, Yuodelis R A, Page R C. *Periodontal Disease.* pp 392–395. Philadelphia: Lea and Febiger, 1977.

Shore N A. *Occlusal equilibration and temporomandibular joint dysfunction.* Philadelphia: Lipincott, 1959.

Stuart C E. Good occlusion for natural teeth. *J. Prosthet Dent* 1964; **14**: 716–724.

Non-working side contacts

Anderson J A, Isaacson D, O'Bannon J, Wipf H. Consolidation committee report on eccentric relationships. In *Occlusion, the state of the art.* (ed). Celenza F V, Nasedkin J N, pp 142–145. Chicago: Quintessence, 1978.

Butler J, Stallard R. Effect of occlusal relationships on neurophysiological pathways. *J Periodont Res* 1969; **4**: 141–151.

Gilmore N D. *An epidemiologic investigation of vertical osseous defects in periodontal disease.* University of Michigan: PhD thesis, 1970.

Yuodelis R A, Mann W V. The prevalence and possible role of non-working contacts in periodontal disease. *Periodontology* 1965; **3**: 219–223.

Mandibular sideshift

Bennett N G. A contribution to the study of the movements of the mandible. *J. Prosthet Dent* 1958; **8**: 41–54.

Lundeen H C, Worth C G. Condylar movement patterns engraved in plastic blocks. *J. Prosthet Dent* 1973; **30**: 866–875.

Lundeen H C, Shyrock E F, Gibbs C H. An evaluation of mandibular border movements their characters and significance. *J Prosthet Dent* 1978; **40**: 442–452.

Preiskel H. Bennett's movement: a study of human lateral mandibular movement. *Br Dent J* 1970; **129**: 372–377.

Preiskel H. The canine teeth related to Bennett movement. *Br Dent J* 1971; **131**: 312–315.

Tupac R G. Clinical importance of voluntary and induced Bennett movement. *J. Prosthet Dent* 1978; **40**: 39–41.

Occlusal splints

Franks A S T. Conservative treatment of temporomandibular joint dysfunction; a comparative study. *Dent Practitioner* 1965; **15**: 205–210.

Green C S, Laskin D M. Splint therapy for the myofascial pain dysfunction syndrome: a comparative study. *J Am Dent Assoc* 1972; **84**: 624–628.

Ramfjord S P, Ash M M. *Occlusion*. 2nd ed, pp 245–255. Philadelphia: W. B. Saunders, 1971.

Zarb G A, Speck J E. The treatment of mandibular dysfunction. In *Temporomandibular joint function and dysfunction*. Zarb G A, Carlsson G E, (ed). pp 378–381. Copenhagen: Munksgaard, 1979.

Articulators

Celenza F V. An analysis of articulators. *Dent Clin North Am* 1979; **23**: 305–326.

Crispin B J, Myers G E, Clayton J A. Effects of occlusal therapy on pantographic reproducibility of mandibular border movements. *J. Prosthet Dent* 1978; **40**: 29–34.

Dawson P E. *Evaluation, diagnosis and treatment of occlusal problems*. pp 111–145. St Louis: C V Mosby, 1974.

Ramfjord S P, Ash M M. *Occlusion*. 2nd ed, pp 222–229. Phildelphia: W. B. Saunders, 1971.

Shields J M, Clayton J A, Myers G E. Using pantographic tracings to detect TMJ and muscle dysfunctions. *J. Prosthet Dent* 1978; **80**: 39–44.

Shillingburg H T, Hobo S, Whitsett L D. *Fundamentals of fixed prosthodontics*. pp 55–65. Chicago: Quintessence, 1978.

Waxing

Huffman R W, Regenos J. *Principles of occlusion*. pp 211–215. London, Ohio: H and R Press, 1977.

Lundeen H C. *Introduction to occlusal anatomy*. Lexington: University of Kentucky, 1969.

Schluger S, Yuodelis R A, Page R C. *Periodontal disease: basic phenomena, clinical management and occlusal and restorative interrelationships*. pp 684–695. Philadelphia: Lea and Febiger, 1977.

Shillingburg H T, Hobo S, Whitsett L D. *Fundamentals of fixed prosthodontics*. pp 241–254. Chicago: Quintessence, 1978.

Thomas P K. *Syllabus on full month waxing technique for rehabilitation: tooth to tooth cusp fossa concept of organic occlusion*. 3rd ed. Los Angeles: University of California School of Dentistry, 1967.

Registration materials

Millstein M L, Kronman J H, Clark R E. Determination of the accuracy of wax interocclusal registration. *J. Prosthet Dent* 1971; **25**: 189.

Millstein M L, Clark RE, Kronman J H. Determination of the accuracy of wax interocclusal registrations, part II. *J Prosthet Dent* 1973; **29**: 40.

Mullick S C, Stackhouse J A Jr, Vincent G R V. A study of interocclusal record materials. *J Prosthet Dent* 1981; **46**: 304–307.

Strohaver R A. A comparison of articulator mountings made with centric relation and myocentric position records. *J. Prosthet Dent* 1972; **28**: 379–390.

Occlusal adjustment equilibration

Arnold N R, Frumker S C. *Occlusal treatment.* Philadelphia: Lea and Febiger, 1976.

Dawson P E. *Evaluation, diagnosis and treatment of occlusal problems.* pp 71–100. St Louis: C V Mosby, 1974.

Ramfjord S P, Ash M M. *Occlusion.* 2nd ed, pp 271–311. Philadelphia: W. B. Saunders, 1971.

Schluger S, Yuodelis R A, Page R C. *Periodontal disease: basic phenomena, clinical management and occlusal and restorative inter-relationships.* pp 391–404. Philadelphia: Lea and Febiger, 1977.

Stress concentration

Craig R G, El-Ebrashi M K, Peyton F A. Experimental stress analysis of dental restorations: part II, two-dimensional photo-elastic analysis of crowns. *J. Prosthet Dent* 1967; **17**: 292–302.

Craig R G, Farah J W. Stress analysis and design of single restorations and fixed bridges. *Oral Sci Rev* 1977; **10**: 45–74.

Lehman M L, Hampson E L. A study of strain patterns in jacket crowns on anterior teeth resulting from different tooth preparations. *Br Dent J* 1962; **113**: 337–345.

McLean J W. *The science and art of dental ceramics, vol 1,* pp 189–196, 218–226. Chicago: Quintessence, 1979.